Preface

Modern science has contributed extensively to our understanding of the natural event of menopause. Clearly many of the symptoms and signs of menopause are linked to the role of women in our society because it is not easy to work full-time, and be an excellent housewife and a perfect grandmother at the same time regardless of age.

At around age 50, endogenous oestrogen production decreases and in more than 50% of women this decrease generates symptoms such as hot flushes and sweats, as well as sleep disturbances and palpitations. The other 50% or so of women have no such symptoms. In addition, the ultimate loss of vaginal lubrication and lactobacillae may provoke symptoms from the lower genital tract, such as dyspareunia, increased frequency of micturition and susceptibility to recurrent cystitis. Furthermore, an accelerated loss of bone mass occurs within the first years after menopause, which may lead to osteoporosis and subsequent fragility fractures. Our health care system can help. But will we able to help every woman with hormone-related symptomatology? And if so, for how long?

Regrettably, disciplines as diverse as biochemistry, endocrinology, internal medicine, gynaecology, orthopaedic surgery, psychiatry and the social sciences have moved the issues of the climacteric woman into different areas, including menstrual cycles, bones, the cardiovascular system, hormones, hot flushes and positive benefits. Integrated clinical knowledge remains scarce and major individual differences among patients are often disregarded.

Specific women's health care centres have only been established recently and the advantages of an interdisciplinary approach have become evident. Menopause clinics and women's health care centres can facilitate communication and bring knowledge from many sources, such as from nutritionists and physiotherapists, into clinical focus and thus into clinical practice.

Mitigation of menopausal symptoms by hormone replacement therapy (HRT) is established medical practice today in most of the so-called developed world. But we need HRT regimens that are effective, cheap and safe. Both efficacy and the side-effect pattern, such as gastrointestinal discomfort and breast tenderness, badly warrant improvement. We must also be able to guarantee long-term safety, which we cannot do today.

As 80% of women prefer bleed-free regimens this is where development should focus. The vast majority of side-effects are related to the progestogenic compound used, not surprisingly as the commercially available progestogens were targeted for purposes other than oestrogen co-medication in HRT regimens for climacteric women. Only recently, a progestogen has been developed primarily for co-medication with oestrogens. However, extended clinical use will provide the ultimate evidence for efficacy and safety of a new compound.

In the modern, western world a woman can expect to live another 30 years after the menopause, which corresponds to about one-third of her lifetime. One out of six, and soon one out of five individuals, is a woman of postmenopausal age. This figure is equal to the number in a retirement community or all students in a given country, if you combine all educational programmes from primary school up to and including university. These large numbers of individuals constitute a challenge to the ever-decreasing medical resources.

As HRT may positively influence several conditions that postmenopausal women experience, there is an obvious need to disseminate current knowledge, especially outside the field of obstetrics and gynaecology. In the very near future, non-specialists will give advice to most postmenopausal women. While the general principles of HRT are increasingly well known by most physicians, there are many practical considerations that a doctor needs to consider when prescribing HRT for the patient. The impact of pre-existing conditions and pertinent health concerns need to be addressed on an individual basis.

By combining an up-to-date underlying knowledge of pathophysiology with case histories this book aims to highlight the present position of common female health conditions in relation to the use of oestrogens and progestogens.

Abbreviations

AHA	American Heart Association
BMI	body mass index
CHD	coronary heart disease
CVD	cardiovascular disease
CEE	conjugated equine oestrogens
DEXA	dual x-ray absorptiometry
DHEAS	dehydroepiandrosterone sulphate
FAI	female androgen insufficiency
FSH	follicle stimulating hormone
HRT	hormone replacement therapy
LH	luteinizing hormone
MPA	medroxy-progesterone acetate
MI	myocardial infarction
PEPI	postmenopausal oestrogen/progestin interventions
SHBG	sex hormone binding globulin
TG	triglyceride
VTE	venous thromboembolism
WHI	Women's Health Initiative

Contents

Preface	iii
Abbreviations	vi
Introduction	9
Hormonal changes	11
Premature menopause	13
Diagnosis	15
Hormonal evaluation	16
Diagnosis of premature menopause	17
Acute Symptoms of the Menopause	18
Hot flushes	19
Urinary incontinence	22
Urinary tract infection	23
Vaginal atrophy	23
Sexual function	25
Mood, depression and cognitive function	28
Hormone Replacement Therapy – The Agents	30
Use of HRT	30
Oestrogens	30
Progestogens	35
HRT regimens	37
Bleeding problems in HRT users	38
When is HRT indicated?	39
Androgen Replacement	41
Measuring androgens	41
Diagnosis of androgen deficiency	43
Symptoms	44
Using androgen replacement	47
Risks of androgen replacement	48
Available androgen replacement	49
Osteoporosis	51
Estimating fracture risk	54
Effects of HRT on fracture	58
Effects of HRT regimens on bone density	60
Appropriate HRT regimens	60
Timing of therapy	60
Phytoestrogens	61

SERMs 61
Bisphosphonates 62
General measures for the prevention of
osteoporosis 62

Cardiovascular Disease and HRT 64
The HERS study 64
The WHI study 65
Other studies 67
Recommendations 69
Stroke 74
Conclusion 74

Prevention of Alzheimer's Disease 76
Prevention of cognitive decline 76
Reduction in the risk of developing
dementia 77
Treatment for Alzheimer's disease 77

HRT and Cancer Risk 78
Breast cancer 78
Endometrial cancer 84
Risk of endometrial hyperplasia 85
Ovarian cancer 87
Cervical cancer 88
Colorectal cancer 88

HRT and Risk of Venous Thromboembolism 89

Future Developments 93
Oestrogen components 95
Progestogens and progesterone 97

Frequently Asked Questions 100

References 107

Appendix 1 – Drugs 120

Appendix 2 – Useful Addresses and Websites 139

Index 140

Introduction

Menopause – the final menstrual period – marks the end of spontaneous menstruation. Clinically, menopause is determined retrospectively and is diagnosed after 12 months of amenorrhoea (Table 1).

The average age at menopause is 51 years, although it commonly occurs as early as 45 years or as late as 56 years. Most women experience several years of menstrual irregularity and varying menopausal symptoms prior to their final menstrual bleed. The average woman can expect to live for over one-third of her life in the postmenopausal period (Figure 1).

It is likely that age at menopause has a genetic component. Race, use of oral contraceptives, number of pregnancies and age at menarche have not been shown to affect the age at menopause. Smoking, on the other hand, appears to bring forward the age at menopause by 1 or 2 years.[1]

The decline in ovarian function prior to the menopause is associated with a number of acute menopausal symptoms, which are caused by fluctuating oestrogen levels and the lack of oestrogen at menopause (Table 2). However, not all women have these symptoms.

Definition of menopause
Menopause: permanent cessation of menstruation resulting from the loss of ovarian follicular activity
Perimenopause (or climacteric): Period immediately before the menopause with endocrinological, biological and clinical features of approaching menopause, and at least the first year after the menopause
Postmenopause: The stage of life following the date of the last menstrual bleed, which cannot be determined until 12 months of amenorrhoea

Table 1. Definition of menopause.

Longer-term implications of a lack of oestrogen include:
- Reduction in bone density leading to osteoporosis and an increased risk of fracture
- Increased risk of cardiovascular disease (CVD)

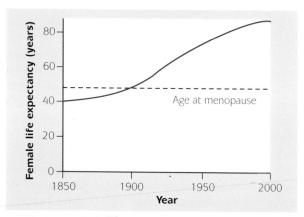

Figure 1. Changing life expectancy. Reprinted from Abernethy K. *The Menopause and HRT*, 2nd edition. Balliere Tindall, copyright (2001),[1] with permission from Elsevier Science.

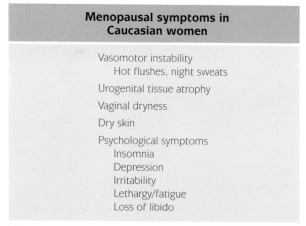

Table 2. Menopausal symptoms in Caucasian women.

Hormonal changes

Ten to 15 years prior to the menopause the ovaries become increasingly resistant to hormonal stimulation. The hypothalamus and the anterior pituitary gland compensate by increasing the release of gonadotropic hormones. Eventually, the remaining ovarian follicles fail to ripen despite continued secretion of follicle stimulating hormone (FSH) and luteinizing hormone (LH), and there is a subsequent fall in oestrogen, oestrone and progesterone.

In premenopausal women, oestradiol and oestrone are secreted by the ovaries. Oestrone is less biologically active than oestrogen and is produced in adipose tissue from androstenedione. Prior to the menopause, levels of oestradiol are higher than levels of oestrone. This is reversed after the menopause because oestrone continues to be produced in adipose tissue (Table 3).

During perimenopause, levels of FSH tend to fluctuate – levels may be raised to the postmenopausal range in some cycles, but return to premenopausal levels in others. Therefore, measurement of FSH levels should not be used to diagnose menopause in those women who are still menstruating. However, measurement of FSH levels can be useful in the following circumstances:

Hormonal changes following the menopause	
Hormone	**Change in concentration**
Oestradiol	↓
Oestrone	↓
Progesterone	↓ abolished
FSH	↑
LH	↑
Androstenedione, testosterone	↓
Sex hormone binding globulin	↓

Table 3. Hormonal changes following the menopause.

- In the diagnosis of premature menopause
- After hysterectomy
- To confirm lack of ovarian function and inform contraceptive requirements (Figure 2)

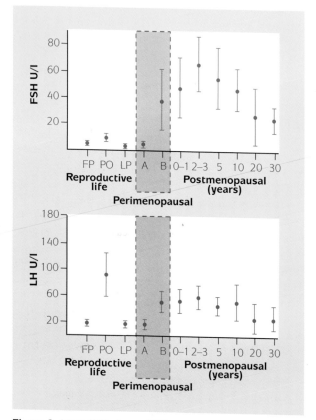

Figure 2. Mean (SD) plasma FSH and LH values in pre-, peri- and postmenopausal women. FP=follicular phase, PO=peak ovulatory value, LP=luteal phase. A and B are women still menstruating with apparent menopausal symptoms, B represents women with vasomotor symptoms. Reprinted from Whitehead M. *Hormone replacement therapy — Your Questions Answered.* Copyright (1992) with permission from Elsevier Science.

Androgen activity

The two most abundant endogenous androgens are androstenedione and testosterone, which are produced by the ovary. Androstenedione is also manufactured by the adrenals. Both steroids decrease after menopause. However, the carrier protein, sex hormone binding globulin (SHBG), is also decreased. The clinical picture may result from increased androgen activity (increased facial hair growth and lowered voice).

Premature menopause

Premature ovarian failure is defined as a syndrome occurring before the age of 40 years and characterized by primary or secondary amenorrhoea, raised FSH and LH levels and low oestrogen levels. Primary ovarian failure occurs when the woman fails to menstruate at all on reaching puberty, and often has a genetic cause.[1]

Secondary ovarian failure is more common and occurs when the woman has experienced normal menstruation, but subsequently experiences amenorrhoea as a result of ovarian failure.[1]

Premature ovarian failure accounts for 2–10% of women with primary or secondary amenorrhoea, and it is estimated that 1–3% of the population is affected.[2]

The cause of premature menopause is often difficult to establish; however, potential causes include:

- Genetic factors. In women with Turner's syndrome the ovaries develop normally, but accelerated follicular atresia causes ovarian failure[3]
- Autoimmune disease (Addison's disease, diabetes mellitus and hypothyroidism)
- Infection with the mumps virus

Surgical menopause

Hysterectomy with oophorectomy is the most common cause of a premature menopause. Removal of the ovaries results in a sudden fall in oestrogen levels (Figure 3) and symptoms may occur very quickly. Women who experience early

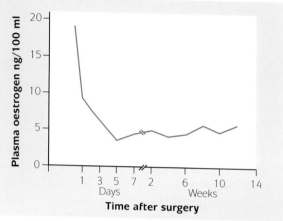

Figure 3. Oestrogen levels after oophorectomy in a premenopausal woman.

menopause as a result of surgery are at a higher risk of osteoporosis and coronary heart disease compared with women who experience menopause around age 50.

Women who have had a hysterectomy with conservation of the ovaries may also experience ovarian failure, as a result of failing vascular supply to the ovaries. Other women who undergo hysterectomy with conservation of the ovaries may experience a temporary phase of menopausal symptoms until their ovaries re-establish function.

Other iatrogenic causes – radiotherapy and chemotherapy

Radiotherapy may lead to ovarian failure. The risk of ovarian failure depends on the age of the patient, the dose of radiation and the length of treatment. Shielding the ovaries during treatment reduces the dose of radiation able to reach the ovaries.[4]

Chemotherapy has an adverse effect on the ovaries in most women. Women aged over 30 years at the time of treatment are likely to experience permanent ovarian failure, whilst those aged under 30 years are likely to experience an early menopause several years after the treatment.[5]

Diagnosis

In general, menopause is obvious from the history and the patient's current symptoms should be carefully assessed. The American Association of Clinical Endocrinologists guidelines (published in December 1999)[6] recommend that the history should include details of the following:

- Detailed chronological reproductive history including age at menarche, gravidity and parity, detailed menstrual history
- History of hormonal treatment – including contraceptives, oestrogens, preogesterone and androgens
- Sexual history
- Any symptoms of pelvic floor relaxation and/or bladder dysfunction
- Bone/joint pain, arthritis, osteoporosis (bone density measurement) and fractures
- Loss of height
- General medical history (past and present), family history (especially of early menopause, heart disease, osteoporosis, cancer and dementia) and social history
- Dietary history (intake of sodium, vitamin D and calcium), weight fluctuation and physical activity
- Medications
- Quality of life assessment, psychiatric history
  A physical examination should include the following:[6]
  - Posture (to assess for osteoporotic vertebral fracture), gait (flexibility), muscle tone and coordination
  - Body mass index (BMI), body composition and waist size
  - Breast examination
  - Pelvic examination
  - Eyesight and hearing (in terms of fracture risk and quality of life)

Hormonal evaluation

FSH levels increase as menopause approaches. In those women who are still experiencing menstrual bleeding (whether cyclically or irregularly), FSH levels on day 2 or 3 after the onset of menstruation are considered to be increased if they rise above 10–12 mIU/ml. Menopause itself is associated with considerably increased levels, usually greater than 40 mIU/ml.[6]

As discussed earlier, FSH levels tend to fluctuate in perimenopausal women and therefore FSH cannot be relied upon to establish the true onset of menopause.

In perimenopausal women taking hormonal contraceptives, FSH and LH are often suppressed, making assessment of ovarian function more difficult. Hormonal evaluation in these women should be carried out after discontinuation of hormonal contraceptives. The patient's clinical response to removal of hormonal contraception should be assessed – in particular the appearance of any menopausal symptoms.

Serum oestrogen levels are variable in the perimenopause and single oestrogen measurements are rarely useful.

Hyperprolactinaemia will suppress gonadotropin levels, therefore prolactin should be measured in women of perimenopausal age and signs of oestrogen deficiency, but who have normal FSH levels.

Determination of serum progesterone is not useful in amenorrhoeic menopausal women. However, in those women who do menstruate, progesterone levels can be used to determine the timing of ovulation.

Determination of serum androgens [testosterone, free testosterone and dehydroepiandrosterone sulphate (DHEAS)] is indicated in women with symptoms of hyperandrogenism. In women who are still menstruating, androgen levels should be measured during the first week of the follicular phase.

Measurement of thyroid hormones is useful to diagnose hypothyroidism, which is relatively common in this age group. Thyroid hormones may also be measured to rule out hyperthyroidism, which can cause hot flush-like symptoms.

Although pregnancy is unlikely during the perimenopause, β-human chorionic gonadotropin levels should be checked if pregnancy is suspected.

Diagnosis of premature menopause

A diagnosis of premature menopause should be considered in any woman with a history of prolonged amenorrhoea, whether or not she is experiencing menopausal symptoms. FSH levels should be measured serially on at least two occasions – however, even persistently raised FSH levels can not be considered as an absolute diagnosis. In fact, some studies have shown that it is possible (although rare) for women with FSH levels above 40 mIU/ml to ovulate and even become pregnant. Chromosome analysis should be considered in women under 35 years.[2]

Acute Symptoms of the Menopause

Figure 4 illustrates the potential acute symptoms of the menopause.

Fortunately, it is extremely rare for one woman to experience all of the symptoms; however, it is estimated that 75% of postmenopausal women do experience some acute symptoms, often starting before menstruation ends.[1] Many symptoms are self-limiting and cause only mild discomfort, but others may cause extreme distress (Table 4).[1]

Acute menopausal symptoms tend to last for around 2 years. The severity and frequency of symptoms is variable (Figure 5), and symptoms may be constant or may come and go.[1]

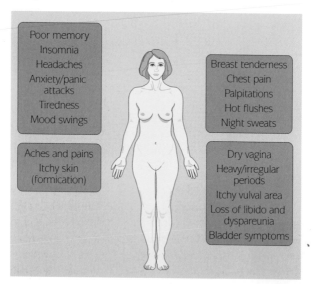

Poor memory
Insomnia
Headaches
Anxiety/panic attacks
Tiredness
Mood swings

Breast tenderness
Chest pain
Palpitations
Hot flushes
Night sweats

Aches and pains
Itchy skin (formication)

Dry vagina
Heavy/irregular periods
Itchy vulval area
Loss of libido and dyspareunia
Bladder symptoms

Figure 4. Summary of typical symptoms associated with the menopause. Changing life expectancy. Reprinted from Abernethy K. *The Menopause and HRT*, 2nd edition. Balliere Tindall, copyright (2001),[1] with permission from Elsevier Science.

Severity of menopausal symptoms
25% of women continue to experience menopausal symptoms for 5 years
5% of women still experience acute symptoms many years after the menopause
51% of symptomatic women describe their symptoms as severe

Table 4. Severity of menopausal symptoms.[1]

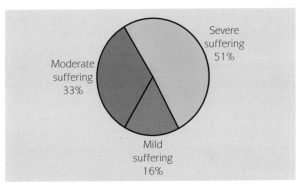

Figure 5. Severity of symptoms in symptomatic menopausal women in the UK. Changing life expectancy. Reprinted from Abernethy K. *The Menopause and HRT*, 2nd edition. Balliere Tindall, copyright (2001),[1] with permission from Elsevier Science.

Hot flushes

Hot flushes are a sensation of warmth, often accompanied by skin flushing and sweating. They may be followed by a chill as core body temperature drops. Hot flushes are thought to be related to the rate of oestrogen withdrawal and the resulting vasomotor instability. The most severe vasomotor symptoms tend to occur in women who have undergone a surgical menopause, as a result of the rapid fall in oestrogen levels.

Hot flushes generally last from 30 seconds to 5 minutes and occur to some degree in most perimenopausal women.[7] One study of perimenopausal women reported that 58%

of women experienced hot flushes in the 2 years around their final menstrual period.[8] Hot flushes can be disabling in 10–15% of women, disrupting sleep, work and daily activities.[7]

There is considerable variation in the frequency and intensity with which women experience hot flushes. Many women experience palpitations, or a sensation of pressure within the head, frequently accompanied by weakness, fainting or vertigo before the flush begins. The palpitations themselves may be a cause of anxiety as some women worry that they may have heart disease. Hot flushes may occur at any time; at night they often manifest as night sweats, causing the woman to wake up feeling extremely uncomfortable. These can continue for months, resulting in chronically disturbed sleep, which may lead to symptoms such as irritability, impaired memory and lack of concentration. Some women also complain of formication (the sensation of tiny insects crawling over the skin), which can be extremely distressing.

Hot flushes may be worsened by hot and spicy foods, alcohol intake, cigarette smoking, caffeine intake and hot weather.

Hot flushes diminish spontaneously as time from menopause increases, although they persist for as long as 6 years.[7]

Treatment

Hormone replacement therapy

HRT is extremely effective against hot flushes.[9] The PEPI (Postmenopausal Estrogen/Progestin Interventions) trial[10] assessed differences between placebo, oestrogen, and each of three oestrogen–progesterone regimens on selected symptoms. PEPI was a 3-year, multi-centre, double-blind, placebo-controlled trial in 875 postmenopausal women aged 45–64 years at the start of the trial. Participants were assigned randomly to one of five groups: placebo, daily conjugated equine oestrogens (CEE), CEE plus cyclical medroxy-progesterone acetate (MPA), CEE plus daily MPA or CEE plus cyclical micronized progesterone.

Symptoms were self-reported using a checklist at 1 and 3 years. In intention-to-treat analyses at 1 year, each active treatment demonstrated a marked, statistically significant, protective effect against vasomotor symptoms (hot flushes) compared with placebo (odds ratios 0.17–0.28). Only those women receiving progesterone experienced breast tenderness.

Clonidine

A small prospective double-blind 8-week trial has shown significant benefit with transdermal clonidine.[11] Of the 15 patients who received clonidine, 80% reported fewer hot flushes; 73% a decrease in severity; and 67% a decrease in duration. Among the 14 placebo-treated patients, 36% reported fewer hot flushes; 29% a decrease in severity; and 21%, a shorter duration (frequency, $p<0.04$; severity, $p<0.04$; and duration, $p<0.03$). However, side-effects of clonidine include drowsiness, dry mouth and dizziness.[7] Other studies have failed to show any benefit.

Progesterone

Megestrol acetate has shown some efficacy in postmenopausal women who have had breast cancer and in men with prostate cancer who have been treated with anti-androgens.[12] A crossover trial of 97 women and 66 men randomized to megestrol acetate (20 mg twice daily) for 4 weeks, followed by placebo for 4 weeks, or vice versa demonstrated that after 4 weeks, hot flushes were reduced by 21% in the group receiving placebo first and by 85% in the group receiving megestrol acetate first ($p<0.001$). An intention-to-treat analysis of data for all eligible treated patients showed that 74% of the megestrol acetate group, as compared with 20% of the placebo group, had a decrease of 50% or more in the frequency of hot flushes during the first 4 weeks ($p<0.001$). Efficacy was similar in men and women and the only side-effect was withdrawal menstrual bleeding in women, generally occurring 1–2 weeks after discontinuation of megestrol acetate.[12]

Vitamin E, Dong Quai and evening primrose oil, all of which are advocated for the relief of hot flushes, were ineffective in randomized controlled clinical trials.

Urinary incontinence

It has been estimated that up to 50% of women experience urinary incontinence to some extent during the menopausal transition period. The lining of the urethra is responsive to oestrogen, and the postmenopausal fall in oestrogen results in physical changes that can increase rates of urinary incontinence (frequency and urgency). Physical changes include: atrophy of the bladder trigone at the base of the bladder, decreased sensitivity of α-adrenergic receptors in the bladder neck and urethral sphincter and thinning of the urethral mucosa.[9] Pain on micturition can be caused by urine coming into close contact with sensory nerves through the thinning urethral mucosa.

Treatment

Pelvic floor exercises and bladder training
Pelvic floor exercises and bladder training can help to alleviate incontinence.[7] A study of pelvic floor muscle exercise in combination with oestrogen replacement versus pelvic floor exercises alone found a significant decrease in stress score in women with mild and moderate urinary incontinence after 3 months of either treatment.[13]

Hormone replacement therapy
A meta-analysis demonstrated that oestrogen replacement had only a positive small effect on urinary incontinence.[14] However, a more recent study found that HRT actually increased incontinence and voiding frequency in postmenopausal women with coronary disease aged younger than 80 years. Included in the study were 1525 women who reported at least one episode of incontinence per week at the start of the trial. Study participants were randomly assigned

to combination HRT (oestrogens plus progesterone) or placebo and were followed for a mean of 4.1 years. Incontinence improved (decrease of at least two episodes per week) in 26% of the women assigned to placebo compared with 21% assigned to HRT, while 27% of the placebo group worsened (increase of at least two episodes per week) compared with 39% of the hormone group ($p=0.001$). This difference was apparent by the fourth month of treatment and was observed for both urge and stress incontinence. The number of incontinence episodes per week increased by an average of 0.7 in the hormone group and decreased by 0.1 in the placebo group ($p<0.001$).[15]

Urinary tract infection

Increased vaginal pH and changes in the vaginal flora at menopause may lead to increased susceptibility to urinary tract infections.[9]

Treatment

Hormone replacement therapy

Oral, transdermal and intravaginal oestrogen may reduce the incidence of urinary tract infections. In one study, 93 women with frequent urinary tract infections were randomized to intravaginal oestrogen or placebo in an 8-week trial. Women in the treatment group had 0.5 urinary tract infections per year, compared with 5.9 episodes in the placebo group.[16] Corresponding improvements in risk factors such as pH and vaginal flora were also seen. Clearly, long-term studies, which show that HRT is the preferred treatment for this condition, are lacking (Figure 6).

Vaginal atrophy

Oestrogen receptors are present in the vagina, and the vagina is extremely sensitive to oestrogen. Declining oestrogen levels lead to changes in the vagina and vulval areas (Table 5).

In clinical practice, women who present to their GP with symptoms of dyspareunia and vaginal dryness, itching and

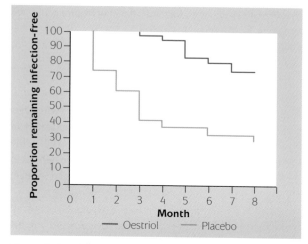

Figure 6. Reduction in urinary tract infections in women receiving oestrogen. Reproduced from Raz R, Stamm WE. A controlled trial of intravaginal estradiol in postmenopausal women with recurrent urinary tract infections. *N Engl J Med* 1993; **329**: 753–759.[16] Copyright © 2002 Massachusetts Medical Society.

irritation often have signs of vaginal atrophy on physical examination. Signs of vaginal atrophy include: epithelial pallor, petechiae, friability and absence of rugae.[9]

Treatment
Hormone replacement therapy
Vaginal atrophy may be treated with systemic or local (oestrogen ring or cream) oestrogen.[9] Usual systemic doses

Changes in the vagina due to oestrogen deficiency
Decreased pH – resulting in reduced resistance to infection
Decreased blood flow
Loss of elasticity
Reduction in length of the vagina
Loss of muscle tone
Decreased cervical secretion/vaginal lubrication

Table 5. Changes in the vagina due to oestrogen deficiency.

should be used, although some women may require additional local vaginal therapy (hormonal or non-hormonal) in the forms of gels/rings if they do not respond adequately to systemic oestrogen.

Vaginal moisturizers

Additional vaginal non-hormonal therapy is sometimes required in those women who do not respond adequately to systemic oestrogen. Vaginal moisturizers (water soluble lubricants such as KY Jelly and Replens) may be helpful in such patients, and are particularly useful in the management of dyspareunia.

A study of 39 women compared 12 weeks of treatment with either Replens or dienoestrol, an oestrogenic vaginal cream. Replens was given three times a week during the 12 weeks of the study, while dienoestrol was administered daily during the first 2 weeks and thereafter three times a week. Vaginal dryness index, vaginal itching and irritation, dyspareunia, pH and safety were evaluated every week for the first month, and every month thereafter. Both treatments significantly reduced vaginal dryness after the first week of treatment, the oestrogen cream causing the most improvement. Symptoms such as vaginal itching and irritation and dyspareunia significantly decreased or disappeared in both treatment groups.[17]

Vaginal moisturizers are an alternative treatment to local oestrogen and may be a useful complement to systemic HRT in patients suffering from vaginal dryness.

Sexual function

There seems to be a trend towards decreased sexual desire and declining frequency of sexual intercourse with increasing age. A US-based survey found that the prevalence of sexual activity was 70% among women aged 45–54 years, decreasing to 60% among those aged 55–64 years.[9] This age-related decrease in sexual behaviour may be influenced by menopause-related symptoms – for example vaginal dryness often leads to vaginal atrophy, which, in turn, can cause dyspareunia. Other commonly experienced changes include decreased sexual desire, diminished sexual response, loss of libido and orgasmic difficulty (Figure 7).

A prospective observational study of 438 women assessed the impact of menopause on sexual functioning. The study enrolled women aged 45–55 years who were still menstruating, and of these, 226 were studied for effects of hormones on sexual functioning. Short Personal Experiences Questionnaire scores indicating sexual dysfunction increased from 42% to 88% during the menopausal period. Mood scores did not change significantly. The study found that the decline in sexual functioning related more to decreasing oestradiol levels than to androgen levels, and that hormone levels were not related to mood scores.[18]

However, it is arguable that non-hormonal factors may have a much larger impact on sexual function during the menopausal transition than changes in ovarian function (Table 6).

Treatment

Hormone replacement therapy

Oestrogen replacement therapy is very successful in the treatment of dyspareunia due to vaginal atrophy.[9] However,

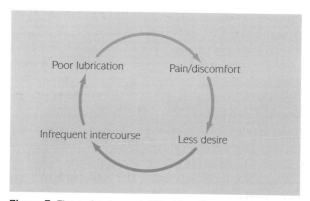

Figure 7. The cycle of sexual difficulties. Changing life expectancy. Reprinted from Abernethy K. *The Menopause and HRT*, 2nd edition. Balliere Tindall, copyright (2001),[1] with permission from Elsevier Science.

Non-hormonal factors that may affect sexual functioning during the menopause
Women's expectation of sexual behaviour/ageing
General wellbeing
Stress
Presence of troublesome symptoms
Feelings for partner
Partner's sexual functioning

Table 6. Non-hormonal factors that may affect sexual functioning during the menopause.

there is some controversy whether other symptoms, such as reduced sexual desire, arousal and orgasm, benefit from oestrogen replacement. However, since oestrogen therapy has beneficial effects on sensation, vasocongestion and vaginal secretions it may also play a role in improved sexual arousal.[9]

The role of testosterone for sexual dysfunction, reduced desire in particular, is controversial. In a randomized trial of 75 women who had undergone oophorectomy, transdermal testosterone (300 µg added to 0.625 mg oestrogen) resulted in improved sexual function as measured by questionnaire.[19] Testosterone replacement is particularly relevant in women who have undergone oophorectomy, since they have significantly reduced testosterone levels.

Psychosexual counselling

Since the causes of menopausal sexual problems are multifactorial, psychosocial counselling may be helpful in some cases. Such counselling is likely to involve:
- Careful and attentive listening
- Provision of information about sexual function
- Reassurance and encouragement
- Suggestions for improving communication within a relationship

In the majority of cases a combination of HRT, counselling and reassurance will be sufficient for a couple to resolve sexual difficulties.[1]

Mood, depression and cognitive function

In addition to physical symptoms, some women experience emotional or psychological symptoms around the time of the menopause. Frequent hot flushes and the resulting insomnia can contribute to these symptoms (Table 7).

Oestrogen receptors are present in the central nervous system; however, it is not known whether declining oestrogen levels contribute directly to the psychological symptoms seen during perimenopause and postmenopause. Midlife is often a time of social and emotional upheaval and there are a number of contributory life experiences that may impact on psychological symptoms (Table 8).

Emotional and psychological symptoms of the menopause that may occur in some but not all women
Depression, anxiety and panic attacks
Emotional liability, mood swings and irritability
Memory loss
Lack of concentration
Decreased or increased libido

Table 7. Emotional and psychological symptoms of the menopause[1] that may occur in some but not all women.

Contributory factors to psychological symptoms
Marriage difficulties and divorce
Children becoming independent and leaving home
Change in responsibility in the home or at work
Death or illness within the family

Table 8. Contributory factors to psychological symptoms.

A number of studies have assessed the prevalence of depression during the menopause. Several report no association between menopause and depression, whilst others report an increased prevalence – up to 51% of menopausal women in one study, particularly in women with a history of depression. It has been suggested that women with previous affective disorders may be at increased risk during the menopause.[9]

Treatment

Hormone replacement therapy

Observational studies have reported some improvement with HRT; however, the results of randomized controlled trials have been inconclusive.[7]

The PEPI trial did not show any improvement in anxiety, cognitive and affective symptoms in the active treatment groups.[10]

Raloxifene

A trial comparing raloxifene (a selective oestrogen receptor modulator), oestrogen and placebo on quality of life in healthy, asymptomatic, postmenopausal women showed very little difference between the three groups. In the multi-centre, double-blind, 12-month study, 398 women were assigned randomly to one of four groups: raloxifene (60 or 150 mg/day), CEE (0.625 mg/day) or placebo. Depressed mood, somatic symptoms, memory/concentration, sexual behaviour, sleep problems and perceived attractiveness were unchanged in all groups. However, mean scores for menstrual symptoms significantly worsened and vasomotor symptoms significantly improved in the oestrogen group and mean anxiety/fears scores improved significantly during raloxifene 60 mg/day administration throughout the treatment period ($p<0.05$).[20]

Hormone Replacement Therapy – The Agents

Use of HRT

HRT is a valid option for women with climacteric symptoms. At present there is a controversy as to whether HRT should be used chronically for prevention to each patient (Table 9).

Oestrogens

Common forms of oestrogen are shown in Table 10.

Route of administration

Systemic oestrogens can be taken orally, or given transdermally, intradermally (patch/skin cream/pellet), vaginally, by injection or via a nasal spray.

Uptake of HRT in female gynaecologists and GPs of menopausal age compared with the general population	
Female gynaecologists	88%
Wives of male gynaecologists	86%
Female GPs	72%
Wives of male GPs	68%
Postmenopausal women aged 54	24%

Table 9. Uptake of HRT in female gynaecologists and GPs of menopausal age compared with the general population.[21]

Common forms of oestrogen (in equivalent doses)
CEE (e.g. Premarin), 0.3–0.625 mg
17β-oestradiol, 1.0–2.0 mg,
Ethinyl oestradiol, 0.02 mg
Transdermal 17β-oestradiol (e.g. Estraderm), 0.025–0.05 mg

Table 10. Common forms of oestrogen (in equivalent doses).

Oral administration

After oral administration of oestradiol, around 70% is immediately converted to oestrone in the liver, yielding a similar E2/E1 ratio to that seen after oral administration of CEE. Oestrone is further metabolized resulting in metabolites with decreasing oestrogen activity; oestriol, which has weak oestrogenic activity, is the most abundant end product. This first pass enterohepatic metabolism leads to variation in oestrogen levels.

Furthermore, the high levels of oestrogen delivered to the liver induce increased synthesis of triglycerides (TGs) and proteins (cortisol-binding globulin, SHBG and angiotensinogen) (Table 11).

Hepatic clearance of oestrogen declines substantially with age. Therefore, a woman of 65 years or older may require only half the dose compared with a woman of 50 years (Table 12).

In theory, the side-effects of oral therapy are reduced if oestrogen is taken with food. This is due to the food-induced increased hepatic blood flow. If taken with meals containing fat (e.g. a fat load – such a glass of milk) a proportion of oestrogen dissolves in the chylomicrons formed by the intestine and oestrogen enters the circulation via the lymphatic system, thus avoiding the first pass effect.

Pharmacology of exogenously administered oestrogens

Oral administration follows first order pharmacokinetics: absorption, during which plasma concentrations rise rapidly, followed by distribution, when the drug is distributed to target tissues and finally elimination. Plasma concentrations vary immensely between individuals, but generally reach a peak 1 to 2 hours after taking the tablet (Figure 8).

The variability in pharmacokinetics between individuals is dependent on:

- Rate of absorption
- Volume of distribution — mainly dependent on the amount of body fat in the case of lipophilic agents such as steroids

Metabolic effects of oral oestrogen

↑ triglyceride levels, ↓ total cholesterol, ↓ LDL-cholesterol,
↑ HDL-cholesterol
↑ Increase cortisol-binding globulin
↑ Increase SHBG
↑ Increase angiotensinogen

Table 11. Metabolic effects of oral oestrogen.

Factors affecting oestrogen metabolism

Liver disease

Impaired intestinal function – decreased bioavailability of
oestrogens

    Malabsorption, diarrhoea

    Fibre-rich diets – oestrogens adhere to fibre

    Use of bulk laxatives – increased faecal excretion of
    oestrogens

Food intake – increased hepatic blood flow leads to reduced
hepatic breakdown

Table 12. Factors affecting oestrogen metabolism.

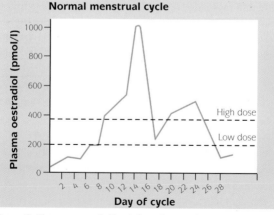

Figure 8. Plasma oestradiol levels (pmol/l) after CEE, 50 μg/day (low
dose) or CEE, 100 μg/day (high dose), compared with levels in the
premenopausal menstrual cycle. Day 1 = first day of menstruation.
Reprinted from Whitehead M. *Hormone replacement therapy — Your
Questions Answered.* Copyright (1992) with permission from Elsevier
Science.

- Rate of elimination — hepatic and renal function, which tend to decrease with age (Table 13)

Topical oestrogen

Gel and cream, have similar pharmacokinetics to those of oral oestrogen, but avoids the first pass effect.

Non-oral oestrogen

Implants, patches, gels and depot injections avoid the first pass effect, which implies a more constant supply of oestrogen compared to oral oestrogens. Nasal spray (300 μg per day), a recent further alternative, differs from both oral and non-oral routes of administration. It is also devoid of a hepatic first pass effect.

Clinical implications

Oral administration is the first-line choice for most women. There is little clinical difference between oestrone or oestradiol in tablets. The hepatic effects associated with oral oestrogens may be particularly helpful in women with hyper-cholesterolaemia, low HDL-cholesterol levels and high levels of homocysteine and Lp(a). However, the long-term clinical impact of the choice of the route of administration in women with the aforementioned constellation of markers is presently unknown.

Non-oral routes of administration may be considered in:
- Women with any hepatic disorder – including alcohol abuse
- Women with a long-lasting disturbance of the enterohepatic circulation
- Women who use bulk laxatives on a regular basis, or with malabsorption
- Heavy smokers
- Users of medication which might interact with hepatic metabolism
- Women with a high TG level.
- Women with hypertension

Factors that enhance/diminish target tissue concentrations after oral administration of oestrogens	
Factors that enhance levels	**Factors that diminish levels**
Alcohol	Smoking
Grapefruit juice	Gastrointestinal malfunction
Drugs	Use of broad-spectrum antibiotics
Cimetidine	Enhanced liver metabolism
Some tranquillizers	Certain enzyme inducers of
Sleeping pills	cytochrome P450 enzyme
Liver malfunction	systems

Table 13. Factors that enhance/diminish target tissue concentrations after oral administration of oestrogens.

Preliminary data appear to suggest that in women with diabetes, pre-stages of type 2 diabetes, hypertriglyceridaemia and migraine, non-oral oestrogen therapy may be a better choice compared with oral preparations. Non-oral delivery of oestrogen does not increase HDL-cholesterol levels.

Non-oral delivery of oestrogen is best avoided in women with skin diseases and/or allergic reactions to the components of patches or creams.

Side-effects of oestrogen

Typical signs of excess oestrogen include breast tenderness, weight gain, bloating and nausea. These are common side-effects at the start of treatment, before a metabolic 'steady state' has become established. Evidence from self-recorded patient diaries appears to show that moderate and severe mastalgia is less frequent with intranasal administration than with oral or transdermal administration. There is considerable inter-individual variation in oestrogenic side-effects. The reasons for this are largely unknown; however, the discovery of more than one oestrogen receptor is an intriguing possibility. Most organs contain both α and β receptors, and the distribution of these receptors may vary from one individual to another.

Interactions with drugs that induce increased activity of the cytochrome P450 enzyme systems in the liver may enhance oestrogen breakdown. Therefore, concomitant medication with cytochrome P450 inducers, e.g. phenytoin, may cause spotting or breakthrough bleeds.

Contra-indications to oestrogen

The true risks of HRT are unknown because women with contra-indications to HRT have been excluded from clinical trials (Table 14).

Progestogens

Progestogens are used to prevent endometrial hyperplasia in women with an intact uterus. The relative risk of endometrial cancer compared to non-users of oestrogen is 2.1 after 2–5 years of oestrogen use and increases to 3.5 after 6 years of use.[22] In the 3-year PEPI trial, over 60% of women taking unopposed oestrogen developed various degrees of endometrial hyperplasia, with 34% developing adenomatous or atypical hyperplasia (Table 15).[23]

Absolute and relative contra-indications to HRT	
Absolute	**Relative**
Active breast, endometrial cancer	Gall bladder disease
Active thromboembolism	Liver disease
Undiagnosed vaginal bleeding	Hypertriglyceridaemia Severe fibroid disease
Active severe liver disease	Previous localized breast cancer
Pregnancy	Previous VTE Untreated hypertension Previous MI
Otosclerosis	Endometriosis

Table 14. Absolute and relative contra-indications to HRT.[1,7]

Progestogens used for prevention of endometrial hyperplasia in combination HRT		
Name	**Cyclical dose**	**Continuous daily dose**
MPA	5–10 mg	2.5 mg
Norethisterone acetate	0.7–1.0 mg	0.25–0.5 mg
Levonorgestrel	75 µg	250 µg
Desogestrel	150 µg	Unknown
Dydrogesterone	10–20 mg	2.5–2.mg tested
Cyproterone acetate	1 mg	Unknown
Natural progesterone	200–300 mg	100 mg
Norgestimate	90 µg	90 µg

Table 15. Progestogens used for prevention of endometrial hyperplasia in combination HRT.

There is no need to prescribe a progestogen in women who have undergone a hysterectomy.

Progestogens used for HRT can be divided into three subgroups
- C-21 derivatives: MPA, dydrogesterone
- C-19 derivatives of nortestosterone: norethisterone acetate
- Natural progesterone and similar compounds

Progestogens differ in their relative metabolic and androgenic effects; for example MPA is minimally androgenic, but does counteract the rise in HDL-cholesterol caused by oestrogen therapy. In contrast, oral micronized progesterone does not mitigate against increased HDL-cholesterol levels. A number of clinical trails have assessed the effect of progestogens on metabolic risk factors; however, outcomes have been inconclusive and observational studies have not confirmed measurable differences in clinical outcomes or metabolic differences.[9]

It has been estimated that 10–20% of women on HRT experience severe progestogen side-effects. PMS-like symptoms are not uncommon and some progestogens may worsen or even induce premenstrual tension. Progestogens have been shown to have an adverse effect on mood in some women, which can be an important reason for non-adherence.

Delivery systems

One of the problems with natural progesterone is its poor oral bioavailability, although, C-21 and C-19 have improved bioavailability. Vaginal creams and the progestogen-containing IUD avoid this problem and deliver progestogens to the uterine endometrium. However, their effect is not confined to the uterus and a systemic effect has been observed. The constant release of progestogen from the IUD is an additional advantage, since it avoids variations in levels.

Tibolone

Tibolone is a synthetic steroid that is structurally similar to norethisterone, danazol and stanozolol. Tibolone has weak androgenic, progestogenic and oestrogenic effects. It appears to stimulate endometrial growth only to a minimal extent, and appears to be an alternative in postmenopausal women with an intact uterus who do not wish to experience a withdrawal bleed. However, tibolone causes increases in LDL-cholesterol and decreases in HDL-cholesterol.[24] To date, it has been difficult to draw firm conclusions as to the benefit of tibolone, since there is a lack of epidemiological data and larger comparative studies.

HRT regimens

The options for endometrial protection are shown in Table 16.

Options for endometrial protection
Cyclical - Sequential progestogen for 10–14 days each month
Continuous combined – daily dose
Intermittent – every 3 months
Intrauterine progestogen

Table 16. Options for endometrial protection.

Commonly used cyclical HRT

- CEE 0.625 mg daily, with MPA 5 or 10 mg on days 1–10/14 of each month
- 17-β-oestradiol 2 mg or transdermal oestradiol 50 μg and a progestogen (Table 15)
- Withdrawal bleeding will occur monthly after day 10/14
- Premenstrual-like symptoms are more common with cyclical HRT

Low dose cyclical oral HRT

- CEE 0.3 mg daily, with MPA 5 mg on days 1–10 of each month if needed
- 17-β-oestradiol 1 mg or transdermal oestradiol 25 μg and progestogen (Table 15)
- Low dose HRT may be sufficient to treat hot flushes in some women

Commonly used continuous combined HRT

- CEE 0.625 mg orally daily, with MPA 2.5 mg orally daily
- 17-β-oestradiol 1 or 2 mg and a progestogen (Table 15)
- Spotty, unpredictable withdrawal bleeding occurs, but usually abates after 6–8 months because of endometrial atrophy

Bleeding problems in HRT users

Other causes of bleeding, e.g. cervical and endometrial cancer, fibroids, endometritis and coagulation disorders, should be ruled out.

With advancing age women may have difficulties in recognizing vaginal bleeding as coming from the vagina. Therefore, if a source of bleeding from within the vagina or uterus cannot be established, examination should rule out a bleeding source in the kidneys, ureters, bladder and urethra and colon or rectum.

Cyclical regimens

Cyclical regimens trigger a light bleed of between 3 and 5 days' duration. However, bleeding may be longer or heavier, and spotting and intramenstrual bleeding may occur. Endogenous production of oestrogens in perimenopausal women increases endometrial proliferation, which leads to heavier withdrawal bleeds. In such cases the oestrogen dose should be reduced to minimize endometrial growth. However, this may result in the return of menopausal symptoms, and increasing the length of the progestogen period may be more helpful.

Continuous combined regimens

Continuous combined regimens are intended not to cause vaginal bleeds. However, during the first 3–6 months of treatment irregular bleeds and spotting is not uncommon, although less so in postmenopausal women. The situation is aggravated if endogenous oestrogens are still being produced. Changing from one preparation to another will seldom correct the problem, even if this change includes a different oestrogen, progestogen or a different mode of administration.

If bleeding problems continue for longer than 6–8 months, or resume even after discontinuation of a continuous combined regimen, then diagnostic tools should be implemented, including an endometrial biopsy to check for potential malignancy.

When is HRT indicated?

There is compelling evidence to suggest that HRT is highly effective in reducing vasomotor symptoms such as sweats and hot flushes. If such symptoms impact on quality of life then HRT is the method of choice for mitigation of these problems. The same holds true for vaginal atrophy and symptoms related to this condition.

Other indications may well exist in individual women but one can never guarantee that, for example, joint pain, sleep problems or incontinence would be significantly improved by HRT. Osteoporosis prevention is a classic indication but given the results of the WHI trial it would seem prudent to use other pharmacologic as well as non-pharmacologic approaches to this condition as treatment probably will continue beyond 4–5 years.

Dosing of HRT is another problem. Unfortunately we have no reliable tools to single out the appropriate dose for a given individual. Plasma concentrations of various hormones are of little clinical relevance to the prescriber and a trial and error situation often occurs. This should follow general pharmacologic principles, i.e. commence with a low dose and, if insufficient, gradually increase the dose. It takes approximately 2–3 months to reach a steady-state condition and it is not relevant to change the dose at shorter intervals if the patient does not have severe side-effects.

It is essential to discuss this with the patient and also to mention that breast tenderness and slight nausea are common during the first few months of treatment. However, these symptoms generally disappear and could be minimized if tablets are ingested with a meal.

It is essential that the patients are given extensive information on the pros and cons of using HRT as this will increase adherence. Apart from clinical examinations including breast examinations, no specific laboratory tests are indicated if the patient feels well. Blood pressure measurements should be taken annually and a mammography performed at least biannually.

One of the most common problems is bleeding discomfort. If this does not readily subside when altering the regimen an endometrial biopsy is indicated. Ultrasonography cannot rule out uterine malignancy or predict endometrial histology.

Women with concomitant disorders that might interfere with oestrogen pharmacology are best referred to a specialist. This is true also for women with a past history of malignancy or diabetes, or those at high risk of cardiovascular disease (CVD), including thromboembolism.

Women on HRT will generally not experience classic climacteric symptoms. It is therefore not self evident when HRT treatment should cease. As a rule of thumb, therapy should preferably not be extended beyond 4–5 years unless severe symptoms reappear when HRT is discontinued.

Therapy could be stopped at any time and if significant symptomatology does not reappear there is generally no reason to restart HRT.

Androgen Replacement

Female androgen insufficiency (FAI) is a relative, rather than a definite, androgen deficiency.[25] The androgens, testosterone and androstenedione, continue to be secreted by the postmenopausal ovary; however, levels are lower than in premenstrual women. In women undergoing oophorectomy testosterone levels fall by 50%, and in these women androgens are only produced by the adrenal gland (Table 17).

Levels of total testosterone decline very gradually with age and may not be noted to be low until women reach their 70s; androstenedione levels decrease much earlier. Levels of DHEAS decline as a function of age and seem to be unaffected by menopausal or oestrogen status.

After menopause, SHBG levels decline slightly, which results in somewhat higher levels of unbound, or free, testosterone (also calculated as a free-testosterone index). The reduction in SHBG reflects reductions in oestradiol and an increase in BMI. However, because of the wide range in values for testosterone and unbound testosterone in perimenopausal women on an individual basis, it may not be possible to predict that a woman may have low levels (Figure 9).

Measuring androgens

Part of the difficulty in determining whether androgens are normal, increased or decreased is related to the variability in measurements. Although the radioimmunoassay for DHEAS is reasonably consistent, upper ranges in women vary between laboratories. Values for increased levels have been reported to be as high as 4 μg/ml. However, one major problem is the weak correlation between symptoms allegedly due to androgen deficiency and peripheral androgen concentrations.

Even greater inconsistency occurs for measurements of testosterone. Methods used vary substantially, and even the use of standardized methods such as radioimmunoassay are variable

Plasma steroid levels in healthy women

	Women of reproductive age	Women after natural menopause	Oophorectomized women
Oestrone (pg/ml)	50 ± 15	30 ± 5	20 ± 3
Oestradiol (pg/ml)	40 ± 3	15 ± 2	10 ± 2
Testosterone (ng/dl)	40 ± 3	20 ± 2	10 ± 2
DHT (ng/dl)	30 ± 4	10 ± 2	<5
Androstenedione (ng/dl)	140 ±10	88 ± 11	64 ± 9
DHEA (ng/dl)	420 ± 21	197 ± 43	126 ± 36
DHEAS (μg/ml)	1.6 ± 0.2	0.8 ± .1	0.6 ± .1

Table 17. Plasma steroid levels in healthy women (mean ± standard error) DHT=dihydrotestosterone; DHEA = dehydroepiandrosterone. Reproduced with permission from reference 25.

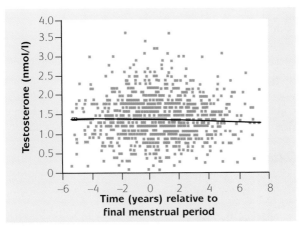

Figure 9. Levels of testosterone pre- and post-menopause. Reproduced with permission from Burger HG, Dudley EC, Cui J *et al.* A prospective longitudinal study of serum testosterone, dehydroepiandrosterone sulfate, sex hormone binding globulin levels through the menopause transition. *J Clin Endocrin Metab* 2000; **85**: 2832–2838.

depending on whether serum is extracted and/or undergoes chromatography before radioimmunoassay. Upper normal ranges vary from 50–100 ng/dl. This makes it difficult to diagnose hyperandrogenism in women with polycystic ovary syndrome and has also challenged the notion of what low levels are in peri- and postmenopausal women. In general, testosterone levels are considered low if they are <20 ng/dl and values are usually below 10 ng/dl after oophorectomy. The most sensitive measurement of testosterone bioavailability is unbound or free testosterone. Tests tend to be unreliable and many investigators prefer to use the free testosterone index, which is a calculated value of the ratio of testosterone to SHBG.

Diagnosis of androgen deficiency

The difficulties in measuring androgens make diagnosis of androgen insufficiency problematic. Androgen deficiency can only be certain in women who have undergone bilateral oophorectomy.

Examples of a relative androgen insufficiency are women with androgen values in the low/normal range and postmenopausal women receiving oral oestrogen replacement, because SHBG levels are increased and unbound testosterone levels are lowered. Additional conditions that may result in relative androgen insufficiency are pituitary adrenal insufficiency, corticosteroid therapy, oral contraceptive use and chronic illnesses, including muscle wasting diseases such as AIDS.

Symptoms

It is important that presenting symptoms occur in a setting that is not explained by systemic or psychiatric illnesses or psychosocial problems, and that oestrogen deficiency has been ruled out (Table 18). Indeed, these symptoms may only be considered to constitute FAI if they persist or worsen, despite adequate oestrogen replacement in a postmenopausal woman. Other cases of chronic fatigue should also be ruled out.

There is a lack of consistent data linking decreased androgen measurements to symptoms. However, testosterone and free testosterone correlate with decreased sexual frequency and desire (Table 19). In a small study, symptoms of decreased sexual arousal and function were more prevalent in women with testosterone levels <10 ng/dl compared to those with levels >30 ng/dl.[26] A decision-making algorithm for iniating androgen therapy in women is shown in Table 20.

Potential symptoms of relative androgen deficiency
Decreased energy and blunted motivation
Flat mood, diminished wellbeing
Irritability, insomnia
Decreased sexual desire or libido

Table 18. Potential symptoms of relative androgen deficiency

Sexual function in women by testosterone levels

Sexual complaint	Low testosterone (<10 ng/ml) n=11	Normal testosterone (> 30 ng/ml) n=11	p	
Decreased desire	11 (100%)	9 (80%)	0.48	ns
Decreased orgasm	11 (100%)	5 (45%)	0.035	
Dyspareunia	6 (55%)	7 (63%)	1.0	ns
Sexual avoidance	9 (80%)	4 (36%)	0.081	ns
Sexual aversion	2 (15%)	0	0.48	ns
Global symptoms	11 (100%)	5 (45%)	0.035	

Table 19. Sexual function in women by testosterone levels.
Reproduced with permission from reference 26.

It should be pointed out that sexual desire and activity in humans are mainly relational and only to a minor extent depend on the hormonal situation.

Decision-making algorithm for initiating androgen therapy in women
Question: Does the woman have symptoms consistent with female androgen insufficiency (e.g. low libido, decreased energy and wellbeing)?
Answer: If yes, initiate evaluation.
Question: Is there an alternative explanation or cause for these symptoms (e.g. major depression, chronic fatigue syndrome, psychosocial problems)?
Answer: If yes, manage as appropriate. If no, evaluate further.
Question: Is the woman in an optimum oestrogen state?
Answer: If yes, continue evaluation. If no, initiate oestrogen replacement.
Question: Does the woman have laboratory values consistent with a diagnosis of androgen insufficiency?
Answer: If yes, continue evaluation. This should include assessment of at least two of three measures of total testosterone, free testosterone, or SHBG. Androgen values should be in the lowest quartile of normal ranges for reproductive age women. If no, consider alternative treatments or referral.
Question: Does the woman have a specific treatable cause for androgen insufficiency (e.g. oral oestrogens, oral contraceptive use)?
Answer: If yes, treat the specific cause (e.g. change medications). If no, consider a trial of androgen replacement therapy.

Table 20. Decision-making algorithm for initiating androgen therapy in women. Reproduced with permission from reference 25.

Using androgen replacement

The concept of using androgen, with or without oestrogen, in women is not new. Early studies mainly looked at methyltestosterone and showed some benefit in menopausal symptoms, general wellbeing and libido.

More recent studies, using testosterone injections or implants, transdermal testosterone and oral methyltestosterone have shown a positive effect on symptoms and wellbeing.[27–31] There is some evidence from these data that the most significant responses are observed in younger women who have undergone bilateral oophorectomy. However, assessment of wellbeing and sexual function is difficult to standardize.

Trials have shown an improvement in parameters of sexual function and wellbeing with testosterone replacement over the use of oestrogen alone. When women use oral oestrogen the increase in SHBG (approximately 75%) results in a substantial decrease in unbound, or free testosterone. A study of women unsatisfied with oestrogen replacement alone found that the women had more energy and less sexual function problems, as well as greater sexual frequency, sensitivity and desire, when testosterone was added to their regimen (Figure 10).[32]

Dose

In oophorectomized women, replacement of oestradiol and testosterone using 50 mg implants (pellets) has been shown to improve wellbeing, sexual function and bone mass.[33] With implants (pellets), testosterone levels tend to be above the normal range (approximately 90 ng/dl), yet lower than with injectable testosterone. A recent study found that a 300 μg dose of transdermal testosterone demonstrated statistically significant benefits in sexual function and wellbeing.[31]

In conclusion, there is some evidence that androgen replacement at near physiological levels may be efficacious for symptoms of sexual function and wellbeing; however, more consistent benefits are achieved with levels that exceed the normal range.

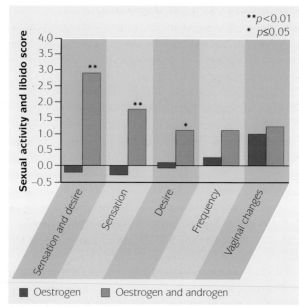

Figure 10. Effect of adding androgen to oestrogen replacement. Reproduced with permission from Sarrel P, Dobay B, Wiita B. Estrogen and estrogen-androgen replacement in postmenopausal women dissatisfied with estrogen only therapy, sexual behavior and neuroendocrine responses. *J Reprod Med* 1998; **43**: 847–856.

Risks of androgen replacement

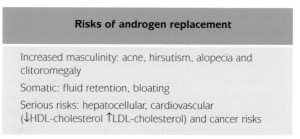

Risks of androgen replacement
Increased masculinity: acne, hirsutism, alopecia and clitoromegaly
Somatic: fluid retention, bloating
Serious risks: hepatocellular, cardiovascular ($\downarrow$HDL-cholesterol $\uparrow$LDL-cholesterol) and cancer risks

Table 21. Risks of androgen replacement.

Available androgen replacement

Various androgen preparations are potentially available for use in women, although these preparations are not presently licensed for use in women. Therefore women in need of androgen replacement should be referred to a specialist (Table 22).

Injected testosterone is not recommended because of varying plasma levels and the risk of steroid accumulation. However, intramuscular testosterone has been shown to be efficacious in oophorectomized women.

Methyl- or fluorinated testosterone in large doses (as used occasionally by men) should not be used. In lower doses methyltestosterone (1.25–2.5 mg) with esterified oestrogens has been shown to be beneficial for menopausal symptoms, bone mass and possibly sexual function and quality of life variables.

Testosterone implants, or pellets (50 mg), are inserted at 4–6 monthly intervals. Monitoring is mandatory and testosterone levels should be obtained before a repeat insertion. Although values vary considerably among subjects, values remain fairly constant for each individual. Values are usually at the upper level of the normal range 70–90 ng/dl.

The transdermal patch (150 µg or 300 µg) has not been approved as yet for use in women. Efficacy in short-term studies has been shown for the larger dose (300 µg) and values are generally in the physiological range with no adverse findings.

Testosterone gel has been approved for men at a 5 mg dose, which provides physiological replacement with steady state levels of approximately 600 ng/dl. By extrapolation, the dose required in women would be less than 1 gm/day (approximately 0.7 gm).

Oral micronized DHEA has been used in various clinical trials. Although it is not the most efficient or efficacious way to deliver testosterone, this approach is an option since testosterone levels are doubled. Because DHEA can lower HDL-cholesterol levels and potentially affect hepatic function, consideration may be given to deliver DHEA vaginally or transdermally. An appropriate oral dose is 25–50 mg daily.

Available androgen replacement regimens	
Method	**Dose**
Injectible (IM) approximately every 4 weeks	
Nandrolone decenoate	25–50 mg
Mixed testosterone esters	50–100 mg
Testosterone enanthate	25–50 mg
Testosterone cyprionate	25–50 mg
Oral (daily)	
Methyltestosterone	1.25–2.5 mg
Testosterone undecenoate	40–80 mg
Subcutaneous and transdermal	
Testosterone implant	50 mg every 4–6 months
Transdermal	150–300 µg every 3.5 days
Testosterone gel	1 mg/day
Other options	
DHEA (oral)	25–50 mg/day
Other androgens (Androstenedione, DHT)	
Other routes (Vaginal, sublingual and buccal)	

Table 22. Androgen replacement potentially viable for women.

Osteoporosis

Oestrogens have important actions on the skeleton at the molecular, cellular and tissue level.[33] Oestrogens regulate fusion of the epiphyses and thus growth in childhood, increase bone strength throughout puberty and protect against loss of bone mineral beyond adolescence. Oestrogen deficiency is a major factor in bone loss after menopause and oophorectomy.

Osteoporosis is the result of substantial impairment of the microarchitecture of bone, both quantitatively and qualitatively, leading to fragility fractures after minimal trauma.

Peak bone mass is achieved by early adulthood and is largely genetically predetermined. Race is an influencing factor; for example, black women have higher bone mineral density than white or Asian women. The development of osteoporosis is dependent on peak bone mass, and also the rate of bone loss at menopause. Around menopause the rate of bone loss is 2% per year for the 5–10 years after the menopause. Early menopause is linked with low peak bone mass and accelerated bone loss (Figures 11 and 12).

Osteoporosis is present according to the World Health Organisation definition if bone mineral density is more than 2.5 standard deviations below the mean normal value for young women (T-score <-2.5).[34, 35]

Osteoporotic fracture – usually manifested as fracture of the hip, wrist (Colles) or vertebrae – is extremely common (Figure 13).

Epidemiological studies suggest that the lifetime risk of a hip fracture for Caucasian women is 17%.[36] Women have a two- to three-fold greater incidence of vertebral fractures than men – this is due to increased bone loss and number of falls (Figure 14).

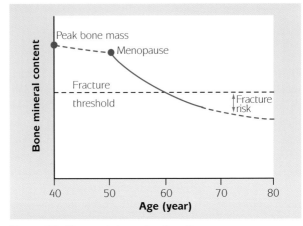

Figure 11. Changes in bone density with age.

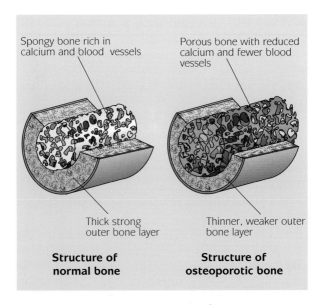

Figure 12. Structure of normal and osteoporotic bone.

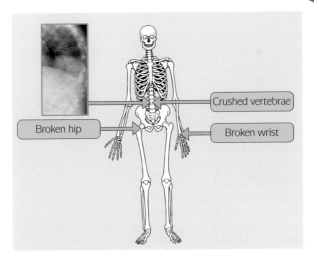

Figure 13. Common sites for osteoporotic fractures.

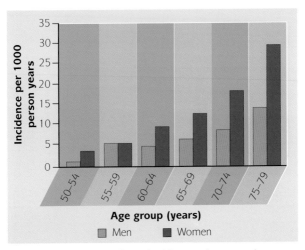

Figure 14. Prevalence of vertebral fracture in men and women by age group. Reproduced from Cummings SR, Melton LJ. Epidemiology and outcomes of osteoporotic fracture. *Lancet* 2002; **359**: 1761–1767.[36] With permission from Elsevier Science.

The incidence of osteoporotic fracture is increasing; this is primarily due to the increase in life span.[36] There is some indication that age-adjusted fracture incidence has increased approximately two-fold over the last 50 years.[37]

Osteoporosis has a considerable impact on morbidity and mortality. The effect of fractures on survival is dependent on the site of the fracture – with hip fracture being the most serious. The risk of death is greatest immediately after the fracture and decreases over time (Figure 15).

Estimating fracture risk

Osteoporosis is present well before the clinical presentation of a fracture. Clinical signs prior to fracture include loss of height and kyphosis (Dowager's Hump).

Fracture risk can be estimated based on bone density (measured by dual x-ray absorptiometry [DEXA]) and clinical factors. Quantitative ultrasound plays an increasing role in

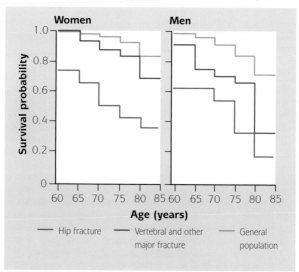

Figure 15. Cumulative survival probability by type of fracture and sex. Reproduced from Cummings SR, Melton LJ. Epidemiology and outcomes of osteoporotic fracture. *Lancet* 2002; **359**: 1761–1767.[36] With permission from Elsevier Science.

the assessment of fracture risk. The risk of fracture is inversely proportional to bone mineral density, and it is far more accurate to measure bone density to predict fracture risk, than to rely on clinical risk factors alone (Table 23).

Measurements of bone mineral density at the lumbar spine and proximal femur using DEXA is the gold standard for diagnosis of osteoporosis (Figure 16). Prediction of specific fractures is more reliable when bone density is measured at that site, e.g. femur for hip fracture.

It is clearly impractical and expensive to scan every postmenopausal woman; however, the following groups benefit from determination of fracture risk by DEXA scan:

- Women at the menopause in whom the decision to initiate HRT would be affected by results
- Women with osteopenia diagnosed on spinal x-ray
- Women on long-term corticosteroid therapy (>7.5 mg prednisolone or equivalent per day)
- Women with a history of one osteoporotic fracture
- Women with a BMI <19 kg/m^2
- Women with an early menopause (surgical or natural) or prolonged amenorrhoea
- Women with a strong family history of osteoporosis
- Women being monitored for response to therapy

Clinical risk factors for osteoporosis
Increasing age
Family history of hip fracture
Previous low trauma fracture
Early menopause
Long-term corticosteroid therapy (>7.5 mg prednisolone or equivalent per day)
Low body weight
Race

Table 23. Clinical risk factors for osteoporosis.

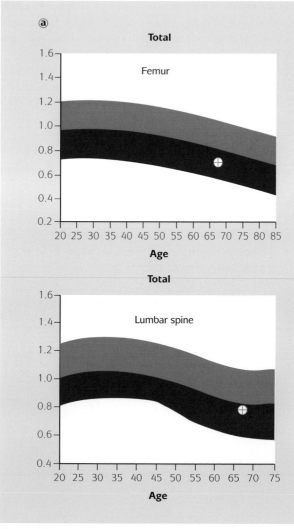

Figure 16. DEXA scan showing low bone density.

ⓑ

DEXA results summary						
Region	Area (cm²)	BMC (g)	BMD (g/cm²)	T-Score	PR (%)	Z-Score	AM (%)
Neck	5.32	2.92	0.548	−3.5	61	−1.4	80
Troch	13.40	6.32	0.472	−2.8	65	−1.3	80
Inter	18.52	15.97	0.862	−2.0	75	−0.6	91
Total	37.24	25.20	0.677	−2.5	69	−1.0	85
Ward's	1.19	0.39	0.325	−4.3	41	−1.4	69

DEXA results summary						
Region	Area (cm²)	BMC (g)	BMD (g/cm²)	T-Score	PR (%)	Z-Score	AM (%)
L1	10.79	6.88	0.637	−2.6	69	−0.9	86
L2	13.14	10.94	0.832	−1.8	81	0.1	101
L3	14.35	12.38	0.863	−2.0	80	0.0	100
L4	14.24	11.13	0.782	−3.0	70	−1.0	88
Total	52.52	41.33	0.787	−2.6	74	−0.4	95

Effects of HRT on fracture

Oestrogen stops bone loss in early, late and elderly postmenopausal women, resulting in a 5–10% increase in bone mineral density over 1–3 years.

Data from randomized controlled trials with fracture as an endpoint are summarized in Table 24. [38]

Randomized controlled trials with oestrogen replacement or HRT with fracture as an endpoint in postmenopausal women

Lufkin EG, Wahner HW, O'Fallon WM *et al*. Treatment of postmenopausal osteoporosis with transdermal oestrogen. *Ann Intern Med* 1992;**117**:1–9.[39]

Therapeutic agent:	Transdermal oestradiol 0.1 mg/day for days 1–21, MPA 10 mg/day for days 11–21
Duration of study:	1 year
Study population:	75 ambulatory women with one or more vertebral fracture and low BMD
Mean age:	65 (55–72)
Primary endpoint:	BMD
Secondary endpoint:	Vertebral fracture
Discontinuation:	11%
Fracture risk (95% CI)	Fracture rate (events/100 person-years): RR 0.39 (0.16–0.95)

Lindsay R, Hart DM, Forrest C *et al*. Prevention of spinal osteoporosis in oophorectomised women. *Lancet* 1980;**2**:1151–1154.[40]

Therapeutic agent:	Mestranolol, mean dose 23 μg in 2 years before analysis
Duration of study:	Median 9 years
Study population:	259 oophorectomized women
Mean age:	48
Primary endpoint:	Coronary heart disease
Secondary endpoint:	Spine score
Discontinuation:	61%
Fracture risk (95% CI)	Spine score: Placebo=1.62 versus mestranol 0.35 (*p*<0.01)

Hulley S, Grady D, Bush T *et al*. Randomized trial of estrogen plus progestin for secondary prevention of coronary heart disease in postmenopausal women. Heart and Estrogen/Progestin Replacement Study (HERS) Research Group. *JAMA* 1998;**280**:605–613.[41]

Therapeutic agent:	CEE 0.625/day, MPA 2.5 mg/day
Duration of study:	Mean 4.1 years
Study population:	2763 postmenopausal women with CHD and an intact uterus
Mean age:	67 (44–79)
Primary endpoint:	CHD
Secondary endpoint:	Hip, non-hip or any fracture
Discontinuation:	11%
Fracture risk (95% CI)	Hip fracture: RH 1.1 (0.49–2.5)
	Non-hip fracture: RH 0.93 (0.73–1.2)
	Any fracture: RH 0.95 (0.75–1.21)

Table 24. Randomized controlled trials with oestrogen replacement or HRT with fracture as an endpoint in postmenopausal women.

Our knowledge largely depends on observational evidence from case-control and cohort studies.[38] One meta-analysis based on trials conducted to assess bone mineral density demonstrated that the use of HRT is associated with a reduction of non-vertebral fractures, in particular in women with uptake of HRT before the age of 60.[44]

Komulainen MH, Kroger H, Tuppurainen MT *et al.* HRT and vitamin D in prevention of non-vertebral fractures in postmenopausal women; a 5 year randomized trial. *Maturitas* 1998;31:**45**–54.[42]

Therapeutic agent:	Oestradiol valerate 2 mg/day, cyproterone acetate 1 mg/day for days 12–21, vitamin D 300 IU/day for years 1–4 and 100 IU/day in year 5, calcium 93 mg/day in placebo group in year 5
Duration of study:	5 years
Study population:	464 postmenopausal women
Mean age:	53 (47–56)
Primary endpoint:	BMD
Secondary endpoint:	Non-vertebral fracture
Discontinuation:	21%
Fracture risk (95% CI)	Non-vertebral fracture (HRT group): RR 0.41 (0.16–1.05)

Writing Group for the Women's Health Initiative Investigators. Risks and benefits of estrogen plus progestin in healthy postmenopausal women. *JAMA* 2002;**288**:321–333.[43]

Therapeutic agent:	Conjugated equine estrogens 0,625 mg and medroxyprogesterone acetate 2.5 mg mg daily versus placebo
Duration of study:	Mean 5.2 years (3.5–8.5)
Study population:	16.608 postmenopausal women
Mean age:	63 (50–79)
Primary endpoint:	Coronary heart disease
Secondary endpoint:	Hip fracture
Discontinuation:	42% HRT, 38% placebo
Fracture risk (95% CI)	Hip fracture (HRT group): HR 0.66 (0.45–0.98)
	Vertebral fracture (HRT group): HR 0.66 (0.44–0.98)

Reproduced with permission from reference 39.

Effects of HRT regimens on bone density

Beneficial effects of oestrogen on bone density have been confirmed by many randomized controlled trials, including studies in healthy women 5–10 years after the menopause,[40, 42] women in their 70s[45] and women with established osteoporosis.[46]

Appropriate HRT regimens

The formulation of oestrogen used, and its route and schedule of administration do not appear to influence its efficacy on bone. Oestradiol (1–2 mg/day orally) and CEE (0.625 mg/day) and 17β-oestradiol (50 mg/day) transdermally all have similar effects. However, recent data suggest that halving the dose has a significant enhancing effect on bone density in late postmenopausal women.[47] Opinion is divided as to whether progestogens have an additive effect to that of oestrogen.

Tibolone has effects on bone density comparable to those of oestrogen.

The combination of oestrogen with bisphosphonates and fluoride results in greater increases in bone density than are induced by the individual medications alone. However, it is not known whether this translates into fewer fractures at old age.

Timing of therapy

The finding that bone mineral density can be maintained at a premenopausal level with oestrogen replacement if initiated within the first 5–10 years after menopause, led to the belief that the administration of oestrogens until old age is effective against bone loss. However, the Framingham study could not demonstrate positive effects on BMD in women above the age of 75,[48] and results from another cohort study suggest that bone loss continues in current users of oestrogens aged over 70 years.[49]

Initiation of therapy after age 60 probably produces nearly comparable benefits compared with starting HRT in the early postmenopause,[50] and the shorter time of oestrogen exposure may be associated with a reduced risk of breast cancer.

Until recently, it was suggested that the bone preserving effects of oestrogens wore off after therapy ceased. However, a recent 4-year, follow-up investigation of the PEPI trial did not find accelerated bone loss after discontinuation of HRT.[51] The risks and benefits of long-term HRT for osteoporosis are shown in Table 25.

Risks and benefits of long-term HRT for osteoporosis in postmenopausal women		
Degree of evidence	**Benefits**	**Risks**
Strong	Relief of menopausal symptoms Prevention of bone loss	Vaginal bleeding Breast tenderness Deep vein thrombosis and pulmonary embolism
Moderate	Prevention of fractures	Increased risk of breast cancer after long-term use
Weak	Improvement in cognitive function and prevention of Alzheimer's disease	Slightly increased risk of endometrial cancer Slightly increased risk of ovarian cancer

Table 25. Risks and benefits of long-term HRT for osteoporosis in postmenopausal women. Reproduced with permission from reference 52.

Phytoestrogens

Phytoestrogens are found in many plants and have variable oestrogen-like actions. At present, phytoestrogens are in pre-clinical testing, and to date they do not have a role in the prevention and treatment of postmenopausal osteoporosis.

Selective Estrogen Receptor Modulators (SERMs)

SERMs act as oestrogen agonists or antagonists dependent on the target tissue. Raloxifene inhibits the action of oestrogen in the breast and endometrium, but acts as an agonist on bone and lipid metabolism.

Raloxifene maintains bone density and reduces fracture risk in postmenopausal women. A large, prospective, placebo-controlled clinical trial demonstrated that the relative risk of vertebral fractures is reduced by 30% in women with prevalent fracture and low bone density, and by 50% in women with very low bone density, without fracture.[53] A substantial reduction in the incidence of oestrogen-receptor positive breast cancer has been observed in patients receiving raloxifene.

Raloxifene increases the risks of thromboembolic disease to the same extent as HRT. Hot flushes and leg cramps have been reported as side-effects.

Bisphosphonates

Bisphosphonates inhibit the resorption of bone by osteoclasts. Randomized prospective placebo-controlled clinical trials show that alendronate and risedronate increase lumbar spine bone density, and reduce the risk of hip, vertebral and forearm fractures by up to 56% (alendronate) and 63% (risedronate). Their effectiveness exceeds that of HRT if evidence from randomized controlled clinical trials is given first priority.

However, bisphosphonates may cause upper gastro-intestinal irritation and special instructions for use need to be followed. Bisphosphonates should be taken fasting with a glass of water and the woman should remain upright after intake.

General measures for the prevention of osteoporosis

General measures for the prevention of osteoporosis include:
- Stop smoking
- Maintain body weight (e.g. >60 kg in women of average height)
- Encourage regular weight-bearing and muscle-strengthening exercise to reduce the risk of falls and fractures
- Maintain calcium intake (at least 700 mg/day)

Anti-fracture efficacy of treatments for postmenopausal osteoporosis in addition to the effects of calcium or vitamin D, or both, as derived from placebo-controlled randomized trials		
Drug	**Vertebral fracture**	**Non-vertebral fracture**
Hormone replacement therapy (evidence mainly from observational studies)	± *	± *
Raloxifene	+++	0
Bisphosphonate (alendronate)	+++	++
Bisphosphonate (risedronate)	+++	++
Bisphosphonate (etidronate)	+	0
Calcitonin (nasal)	+	0
Fluoride	–	–
Parathyroid hormone (effect on hip fracture not documented)	+++	++
Vitamin D derivatives	–	0

Table 26. Anti-fracture efficacy of treatments for postmenopausal osteoporosis in addition to the effects of calcium or vitamin D, or both, as derived from placebo-controlled randomized trials.[52] +++=strong evidence, ++=good evidence, +=some evidence, ±=equivocal, 0=no effects, –=negative effects. *CEE 0.6125 + MPA 2.5 mg in the WHI trial reduced the relative risk of both hip and vertebral fracture by one third. Reproduced with permission from reference 43 (See also Table 24.)

Cardiovascular Disease and HRT

During the 1990s HRT was increasingly prescribed to postmenopausal women to protect against CVD. It was thought that, since coronary heart disease (CHD) is a major cause of mortality and morbidity in older women, any protective effect conferred by HRT would have an important impact (Figure 17). Indeed, observational studies suggested that postmenopausal women taking oestrogen have a reduction in all-cause mortality of 40–60%, considered to be primarily due to the reduction in CVD.[54–57]

However, the cardioprotective effect of HRT has been challenged following the results of three secondary prevention trials[41, 58, 59] and, in particular, the recently published early reports from the Women's Health Initiative (WHI).[43]

The HERS study

HERS was the first large-scale randomized trial of HRT for the prevention of coronary heart disease. It was a multi-centre

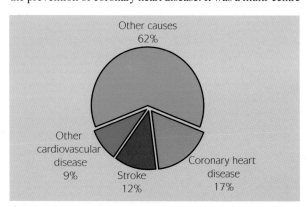

Figure 17. Mortality by cause in women in the UK (2000 data). CVD accounts for 38% of deaths. Reproduced with permission from Peteren S, Rayner M. *Coronary heart disease statistics*. London: British Heart Foundation, 2002.

trial comparing placebo with continuous combined CEE (0.625 mg) with MPA (2.5 mg) in 2763 postmenopausal women (mean age 67) with a history of CVD.[41] The rates of recurrent myocardial infarction (MI) or CHD death were similar in both groups (Figure 18).

The women in the HRT group had significant changes in their lipid profile – by the end of the first year mean LDL-cholesterol levels had fallen by 14% in the HRT group and by 3% in the placebo group ($p<0.001$) and mean HDL-cholesterol levels had risen by 8% in the HRT group and fallen by 2% in the placebo group ($p<0.001$) (Figure 19).

These results have been challenged on the basis of decreased power (shorter follow-up than planned); a lower event rate in the placebo group than that anticipated; and a high crossover rate of women from HRT to placebo.[60] Furthermore, 45% of the women were taking lipid-lowering and other cardiac drugs. Statin use was more prevalent in the placebo group compared with the HRT group. The higher CVD rate in the first year among HRT user was not seen in women who were receiving statins. However, the interaction between statin use and HRT was not significant looking at the overall treatment period of 4.1 years.[61] In further post-hoc analyses, it was apparently not possible to identify subgroups of HERS participants in which HRT was clearly beneficial or harmful. [62]

Recently, follow-up data have been published in the so called HERS-II, the open follow-up study, essentially confirming the results of HERS-I.[63]

The WHI study

The WHI study is a huge study aiming at disclosing the relevance of sex steroids for female health. One part of WHI is a randomized trial on primary prevention of CVD using the same preparation as in HERS but also including an oestrogen-only arm, i.e. CEE 0.625 mg daily. In May 2002, the safety board of WHI decided to discontinue the continuous combined arm as risks exceeded benefits. The results have recently been published in the Journal of the American

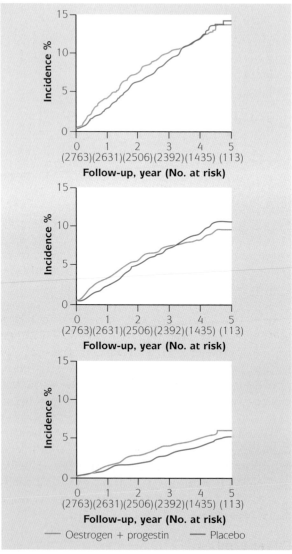

Figure 18. Kaplan-Meier estimates of the cumulative incidence of primary CHD (top), non-fatal MI (centre) and CHD death (bottom). The numbers in brackets indicate the number of women free of an event in each year of follow-up. Reproduced with permission from reference 41.

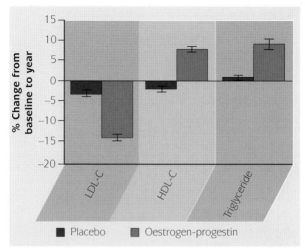

Figure 19. Mean changes in the lipid profile during the first year of the HERS study, expressed as mean changes plus SEM. Reproduced with permission from reference 41.

Medical Association.[43] In essence, the negative results on cardiovascular prevention from HERS were also confirmed in a primary preventive setting (Table 27). The study also confirmed the increased risk of, and also provided further proof for, the prevention of osteoporotic fractures as well as colorectal cancer. The oestrogen-only arm of WHI continues.

In October, the WISDOM study was stopped. This was the second largest placebo-controlled study, with identical trial medications to WHI, that studied the long-term benefits and risks of unopposed CEE and combined CEE and MPA. The Medical Research Council felt that significant results contributing to the field could not be expected anymore; hence the trial was stopped.

Other studies

A 3-year angiographic study found no difference in the progression of atherosclerosis in women with significant coronary heart disease receiving placebo, CEE 0.625 mg or CEE 0.625 mg plus MPA 2.5 mg.[58] The study also failed to

WHI Study. Absolute risks per 10,000 women per year of HRT use		
Clinical Events	CEE 0.625 mg + MPA 2.5 mg daily	Placebo
Risks		
CHD	37	30
Stroke	29	21
Venous thromboembolism	34	16
Breast cancer	38	30
Benefits		
Hip fracture	10	15
Colorectal cancer	10	16

Table 27. Results from WHI study. Reproduced with permission from reference 43.

Clinical CV events and death according to treatment group (Some patients had more than one event)			
Event	Oestrogen (n=100)	Oestrogen + MPA (n=104)	Placebo (n=105)
Death due to CHD	4 (4%)	2 (2%)	3 (3%)
Fatal MI	1 (1%)	1 (1%)	1 (1%)
Non-fatal MI	6 (6%)	6 (6%)	7 (7%)
Any CHD event	29 (29%)	28 (27%)	34 (32%)

Table 28. Clinical CV events and death according to treatment group. Some patients had more than one event. Reproduced with permission from reference 58.

show any difference in clinical CV events and death during the 3.2 year follow-up period (Table 28). A 4-year prospective secondary prevention trial[59] demonstrated similar rates of unstable angina, MI or death in controls and women using transdermal oestradiol with sequential norethindrone acetate.

Recommendations

The American Heart Association (AHA) has issued recommendations regarding HRT and the prevention of CVD (Table 29).[64]

Summary recommendations from the American Heart Association for HRT and CVD

Secondary prevention

HRT should not be initiated for the secondary prevention of CVD.

The decision to continue or stop HRT in women with CVD who have been undergoing long-term HRT should be based on established non-coronary benefits and risks and patient preference.

If a woman develops an acute CVD event or is immobilized while undergoing HRT, it is prudent to consider discontinuance of the HRT or to consider venous thromboembolism (VTE) prophylaxis while she is hospitalized to minimize risk of VTE associated with immobilization. Reinstitution of HRT should be based on established non-coronary benefits and risks, as well as patient preference.

Primary prevention

Daily continuous combined CEE 0.625 mg + MPA 2.5 mg seems not to confer primary prevention of heart disease but firm clinical recommendations for primary prevention await the results of other ongoing randomized controlled clinical trials.

There are insufficient data to suggest that HRT should be initiated for the sole purpose of primary prevention of CVD. Initiation and continuation of HRT should be based on established non-coronary benefits and risks, and patient preference.

Table 29. Summary recommendations from the American Heart Association for HRT and CVD. Reproduced with permission from reference 64.

There is some evidence that women who receive HRT behave in a different way to non-users. It has been suggested that HRT-users tend to be more focused on their health, and may have improved diet and increased exercise levels, which may have a beneficial influence on their coronary risk factors.

If women with established coronary disease do not benefit from oestrogen, then supportive data should exist to show the decreased effectiveness of oestrogen in older women with existing disease. Indeed, several studies have shown that compared to younger women and those without existing disease or risk factors, the effects of oestrogen are diminished or absent in older women with disease. One potential explanation for the lack of a direct effect of oestrogen in older women with diseased vessels is that methylation of the oestrogen receptor gene occurs with ageing and in disease. Therefore, in women with established disease, while it is probable that oestrogen will improve the lipid profile by increasing HDL-cholesterol and decreasing LDL-cholesterol, there are no acute beneficial effects. The beneficial changes in lipid and lipoproteins in women with established disease are unlikely to be able to influence hard endpoints such as MI. Furthermore, these effects are likely to be further overshadowed in those women who use statins.

In the HERS trial,[41] there was a statistically significant increase in cardiovascular events in women with established CVD who started oestrogen therapy in the first year of the trial. In one observational study the incidence of unstable angina was significantly increased in women who began oestrogen in the first year after an event, although mortality was not affected in this study.[65] However, the increased incidence was only seen in new users of oestrogen. In current and past users, the new event rate was not increased, and mortality was significantly reduced in the oestrogen users (Figure 20).

In the Nurses' Health Study, women with established disease who began oestrogen within a year of an event showed a trend for increased event rates, which was not statistically

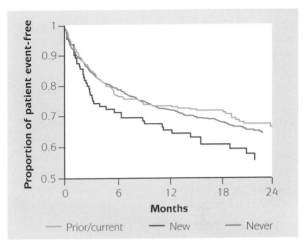

Figure 20. Cumulative incidence of death/recurrent MI/unstable angina requiring hospitalization. Reprinted with permission from the American College of Cardiology Foundation Journal of the American College of Cardiology 2001; **38**: 1–7.[65]

significant in the first year.[66] Again, there was an overall reduction in events after several years of observation.

It remains uncertain why there appears to be early harm in women who initiate hormone treatment within 1–2 years of sustaining a cardiovascular event. Possibilities include the effects of oestrogen on underlying thrombosis risk, plaque instability and inflammation. It is clear, however, that this acute risk is far less likely to occur if a woman is already on a statin, which is known to provide plaque stability and to prevent inflammatory changes.

The results of the WHI study, which was terminated early, at 5.2 years, showed no benefit of continuous CEE 0.625 mg with MPA 2.5 mg when compared with placebo (HR 1.22 (1.09–1.36)). There was no significant time trend within the 5.2 years regarding CHD and stroke, and these effects appeared mainly in the early 1–2 years of the trial (Figure 21 and Table 30). While these results were surprising in that the WHI study

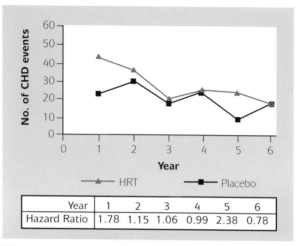

Figure 21. WHI: absolute numbers of CHD events/year/ treatment group. Adapted using data from ref 43.

Cardiovascular events in the WHI study

Events	Absolute no (%) HRT	Absolute no (%) placebo	HR	CI	Adjusted CI
CHD	164 (0.37)	22 (0.30)	1.29	1.02-1.63	0.85-1.97
CABG/PCTA	183 (0.42)	171 (0.41)	1.04	0.84-1.28	0.71-1.51
Stroke	127 (0.29)	85 (0.21)	1.41	1.07-1.85	0.86-2.31
VTE	151 (0.34)	67 (0.16)	2.11	1.58-2.82	1.26-3.55
Total CVD	394 (1.57)	546 (1.32)	1.22	1.09-1.36	1.00-1.49

HR = hazard ratio, CI = confidence interval
VTE – venous thromboembolism
% = annualized per cent calculated from average
exposure over approximately 60 months.
Numbers are absolute numbers of clinical events.
Adapted using data from Writing Group for
Women's Health Initiative Investigators. *JAMA*. 2002;
288: 321-333.[43]

Table 30. Cardiovascular events in the WHI study. Adapted using data from reference 43.

was designed to be a primary prevention trial, it is likely that the negative results are similar to those of the HERS trial (secondary prevention) in that the women were older (mean age of 63 years) and were more than 10 years beyond menopause. However, the negative cardiovascular effects appear to be observed also in younger postmenopausal women.

The role of progestogen

Observational trials have not demonstrated any difference in outcome between oestrogen replacement and HRT regimens. While the null effects of the continuous combined oestrogen/progestogen regimen compared with placebo in the HERS study were criticized on the basis of continuous progestogen use, there was no difference between this regimen and oestrogen alone in the angiographic trial.[58] However, this and several other progestogens have a negative impact on HDL-cholesterol, blood flow and carbohydrate tolerance.

As discussed above, the negative effects in the WHI study were with a continuous combined regimen. The study recruited women who should be seen as representative of a healthy postmenopausal population. Only 400 of the 16,608 women who participated in the trial had a personal history of prior CVD. However, as a large proportion of women were in their 60s and 70s, it is possible that "silent atherosclerosis" without overt clinical events may have been quite common in this cohort of women. The results of the WHI arm that compares oestrogen alone with placebo may provide answers regarding the effect of continuous MPA.

Raloxifene

A recent publication from the MORE (Multiple Outcomes of Raloxifene Evaluation) trial[67] indicated that raloxifene did not increase the risk of CVD, and that it was cardioprotective, with a relative risk of 0.60 (95% confidence interval 0.38–0.95), in the subset of 1035 women with cardiovascular risk factors. These early data need to be substantiated.

Stroke

The impact of HRT on stroke is more difficult to assess in terms of risks and benefits. Some observational data have suggested that oestrogen has a beneficial effect on incidence and mortality, whilst other data have failed to show this, including those from the HERS study. One of the studies that did find an increase in risk, suggested that this risk is on the basis of dose.[68] The statistical increase in risk was confirmed only in women using larger doses of CEE (0.625 mg and greater).

The 0.3 mg dose showed a similar coronary benefit and did not increase the incidence of stroke. Once again, the results of WHI using the dose of 0.625 mg with continuous MPA 2.5 mg showed an overall increase in the risk of stroke (HR: 1.41 (1.07–1.85)).

In the WHI study, the hazard ratio was increased in the HRT group: the hazard ratio was 1.20 for fatal stroke and 1.50 for non-fatal stroke.[43]

Conclusion

It is reasonable to conclude that oestrogen has multiple protective mechanisms on the cardiovascular system, which should be expected to translate into beneficial effects on CVD in women. Accordingly, oestrogen may still have a significant role in primary prevention of CVD disease. No such collaborative data exist at present.

However, this does not appear to be the case for older women with established disease, who may or may not have experienced an event. In this setting, unless a woman is already on oestrogen and benefiting from therapy for other indications when she experiences an event, there is no indication to prescribe oestrogen for cardioprotection. On the other hand, established oestrogen users who have an event may be better protected from death.

Recent observational data have suggested the efficacy of using lower doses of oestrogen for cardiovascular prevention. However, today there is a lack of data from large prospective randomized controlled clinical trials with positive disease outcomes; thus the use of oestrogen for primary prevention at any dose level is not warranted at present.

It should be kept in mind that non-hormonal strategies, such as lifestyle changes aimed at weight control and cessation of smoking, are essential for prevention of CVD in women.[69]

Prevention of Alzheimer's Disease

Menopausal women often have a subjective sense of cognitive decline, defined by changes in memory or concentration, and may report improvement in symptoms with oestrogen therapy. Consequently, some investigators have suggested that if decreasing oestrogen levels have a short-term effect on cognition during the perimenopausal period, then long-term oestrogen deficiency may play a role in more significant cognitive decline, such as the development of dementia in some women.[70]

It has therefore been proposed that oestrogen replacement therapy may:

- Prevent cognitive decline in postmenopausal women
- Delay or prevent the development of Alzheimer's disease
- Delay or prevent cognitive decline in women with established dementia, specifically Alzheimer's disease

Prevention of cognitive decline

Studies that have attempted to assess the effect of oestrogen therapy on various aspects of cognitive function in healthy postmenopausal women have substantial methodological problems and have produced conflicting results. Overall, studies do not show a benefit in cognitive functioning with oestrogen therapy.

One systematic review concluded that in women with menopausal symptoms, oestrogen therapy may have specific cognitive effects, especially in tests of verbal memory, vigilance, reasoning and motor speed.[71] However, the study acknowledged that it was difficult to separate out these effects from the reduction in menopausal symptoms, such as hot flushes. A number of other studies have failed to show a benefit.[72, 73] A subsequent report from the HERS study, described a lack of improvement in various tests of cognitive function and an actual decrease in physical functional capacity in women largely without vasomotor symptoms.[74]

Reduction in the risk of developing dementia

Studies have also assessed whether oestrogen replacement reduces the risk of developing dementia, specifically Alzheimer's disease. A meta-analysis of case-control studies and prospective cohort studies found a 29% decreased risk for developing dementia among oestrogen users;[75] however, the individual studies were susceptible to confounding and adherence bias and the results of the trial cannot be regarded as reliable. Another meta-analysis of observational studies has suggested a decreased risk of Alzheimer's disease, but again there were limitations in the studies included in the meta-analysis.[71]

Two multi-centre prospective, prevention trials are currently underway to answer this question. It is hoped that the Women's Health Initiative-Memory Study (WHIMS) and the Women's International Study of Long Duration Oestrogen for Menopause (WISDOM) will provide evidence on the impact of specific oestrogen preparations (and progestogens) in the primary prevention of Alzheimer's disease within the next decade.

Treatment for Alzheimer's disease

A recent multi-centre trial of 120 women with mild-to-moderate Alzheimer's disease found no evidence that oestrogen improved cognitive or functional outcomes over 1 year.[76] These results have been confirmed in a smaller 16-week trial of elderly women with Alzheimer's disease.[77]

Summary

There is no reliable evidence that oestrogen therapy improves cognition in healthy postmenopausal women or women with Alzheimer's disease, or prevents or delays the development of Alzheimer's disease.

Table 31. Summary.

HRT and Cancer Risk

Breast cancer

Breast cancer is the most common cancer in women and is a key contributor to mortality, although this is far outweighed by CVD mortality. At age 50 the overall risk for the diagnosis of breast cancer during remaining lifetime is estimated at 7% (Figure 22).

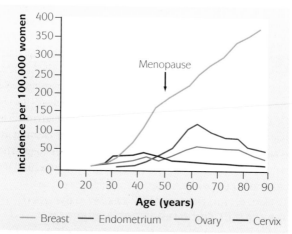

Figure 22. Incidence per 100,000 women of breast, endometrial, ovarian and cervical cancer by age. Reprinted from Whitehead M. *Hormone replacement therapy — Your Questions Answered.* Copyright (1992) with permission from Elsevier Science.

Oestrogen and breast cancer

In observational epidemiological studies, prolonged exposure to endogenous ovarian hormones in the reproductive years (early menarche, late menopause, delayed childbearing and nulliparity) is associated with variable increases in the risk of breast cancer diagnosis later in life. Postmenopausal women with high endogenous oestradiol concentrations are at increased risk, as are women with above average bone mineral density (considered to be a marker of lifelong oestrogen exposure) and increased BMI.

No clinical studies to date have demonstrated that oestrogens initiate human breast cancer. However, the results of case-control and cohort studies have led to concern that exogenous oestrogens after menopause may increase the risk of breast cancer in postmenopausal women.

HRT and breast cancer

A meta-analysis of 51 cohort and case-control studies looked at the relationship between breast cancer risk and the use of HRT.[78] It incorporated 90% of the worldwide literature and re-analysed the original data from 52,705 women with breast cancer and 108,411 control women. It was able to adjust for age at menopause, BMI, parity, family history, alcohol use, smoking history, past combined oral contraceptive use, age at menarche and age when first child was born, but was unable to adjust for differences in breast cancer screening rates. The majority of women were prescribed unopposed oestrogens, mainly CEE (82%), whilst the balance used oestrogen and progestogen preparations. The main findings were as follows (Table 32, Figure 23):

- Current or recent users of HRT had a relative risk of 1.023 (1.01–1.036) for each year of use
- After use of HRT for 5 or more years the risk of breast cancer diagnosis increased to RR=1.35 (1.21–1.49)
- Those who had discontinued HRT at least 5 years previously had no increase in risk

Weight and BMI were shown to modify the relationship between HRT and breast cancer risk, and the increase in relative risk of breast cancer associated with long duration of use was statistically significant only for women with BMI of less than 25 kg/m². The risk of breast cancer in HRT users was not significantly modified by alcohol intake and there was no relationship between type, dose of oestrogen or whether or not unopposed or opposed oestrogen therapy was prescribed. Breast cancers diagnosed in women who had ever

Estimated cumulative incidence of breast cancer

Patient group	Cumulative incidence of breast cancer
Never-users of HRT, aged 50–70	45 per year per 1000 women
Users of HRT, starting treatment age 50, and continuing for 5 years	47 per year per 1000 women
Users of HRT, starting treatment age 50, and continuing for 10 years	51 per year per 1000 women
Users of HRT, starting treatment age 50, and continuing for 15 years	57 per year per 1000 women

Table 32. Estimated cumulative incidence of breast cancer.[78]

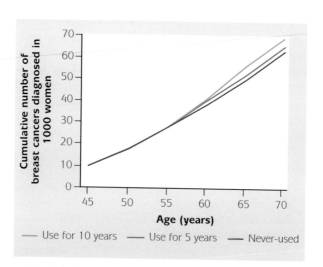

— Use for 10 years   — Use for 5 years   — Never-used

Figure 23. Estimated cumulative number of breast cancers diagnosed in 1000 never-users of HRT, in 1000 users of HRT for 5 years and in 1000 users of HRT for 10 years.[78]
The figure assumes that HRT use began at age 50. Reproduced with permission of Elsevier Science.

used HRT tended to be less advanced clinically than those diagnosed in never-users.

Subsequently, two large cohort studies did not find an increased risk of breast cancer diagnosis associated with the use of HRT in postmenopausal women. In the Iowa Women's Health Study,[79] a large population-based study, 37,105 healthy postmenopausal women aged 55–69 years were followed up for cancer and/or mortality outcomes for up to 11 years, and 1520 incident cases of breast cancer diagnosed. Unopposed oestrogen was not associated with an increased risk either in the short (<5 years) or long (>5 years) term users RR = 1.07,0.94–1.22 and RR = 1.11,0.92–1.35 respectively). The NHANES 1 Epidemiological Follow Up Study was based on participants aged 25–74 at baseline who were interviewed in 1971 and followed for up to 22 years. The incidence of breast cancer was 326/100,000 person years in never-users and 255/100,000 in ever-users of HRT, and no association was found for duration of HRT use.[80] However, this was a study with 219 incident breast cancer cases only.

One Swedish cohort study including 29,508 women (226,611 person-years of observation) and 1145 cases found an increased risk of breast cancer after 4 years of HRT use. [81]

HRT and alcohol use

Alcohol use is one of many environmental factors that may be associated with an increased risk of breast cancer. A pooled analysis of six cohort studies found that the relative risk of breast cancer for women consuming at least 2–5 drinks/day (30–60 g alcohol/day) was 1.41 (1.18–1.69).[82] The analysis found no evidence that the association between alcohol intake and breast cancer incidence was modified by HRT use.

HRT and breast cancer risk in women with benign breast disease

A meta-analysis of studies carried out in the 1980s showed no increase in risk of breast cancer diagnosis in women taking HRT who had a history of benign proliferative breast disease.[83]

Risk of breast cancer with HRT

- Short-term use of HRT (<5 years) is not associated with an increased risk of breast cancer as suggested by the majority of epidemiological data.
- In the Women's Health Initiative oestrogen+progestin trial, breast cancer risk increased after 4 years of use.
- Longer-term use of HRT is associated with a modest increase in risk of breast cancer according to the majority of epidemiological studies.

Table 33. Risk of breast cancer with HRT.

This finding was confirmed by the Nurses Health Study, in which there was no increase in risk of breast cancer diagnosis (RR=1.1, 0.86–1.43) in women with a history of benign breast disease who used HRT, compared to women with no history.[84]

Unopposed oestrogen versus oestrogen plus progestogen

Recent epidemiological evidence suggests that the addition of a progestogen to oestrogen may add to the increased risk of breast cancer. The Breast Cancer Detection Demonstration Project included 46,355 women, representing 473,687 person years, most of whom were receiving CEE and MPA.[85] Increases in breast cancer risk were restricted to those women with hormone use within the previous 4 years, RR = 1.2 (1.0–1.4) for oestrogen-only use and 1.4 (1.1–1.8) for combined HRT.

The results also suggested that oestrogen plus progestogen increases breast cancer risk beyond that associated with oestrogen alone in lean, but not heavier, women. A long-term cohort study of Swedish women found that there was a time-dependent increase in risk after use of combined HRT: the relative risk was 1.7 (1.1–2.6) in women using HRT for more than 6 years.[86]

Recent case-control studies provide further evidence that combined oestrogen-progestogen replacement therapy further increases the relative risk of breast cancer. In one study, the relative risk was 2.43 (1.79–3.30) in women using HRT for at least 10 years, and the odds ratios were always higher in women on combined HRT compared with oestrogen-only therapy in various subgroup analyses.[87]

Three recent case-control studies from the US and Canada found an increased risk of breast cancer with HRT use. In the largest study today, with 5298 cases, the relative risk increases by 2% per year for oestrogen-only, and 4% for oestrogen-progestin therapies.[88] The difference between oestrogen-only and combined HRT was also apparent in a smaller Canadian case-control study.[89] The study by Chen and coworkers suggested that the increase in breast cancer risks may be particularly related to lobular tumours.[90] For a summary see Table 33.

HRT and breast cancer mortality

While the risk of breast cancer diagnosis may be increased in HRT users, it remains uncertain if mortality from breast cancer is also increased. Most studies suggest that ever use of unopposed oestrogen is associated with a decrease in risk of fatal breast cancer compared to non-use.[91] However, conflicting results have been seen in two US cohort studies – one suggesting that HRT does not affect mortality[92] and the other suggesting an increase.[56]

The apparent benefit of HRT on breast cancer mortality appears to attenuate with time[83] and increasing duration of HRT use,[56] and it is not possible to rule out a small increased risk with long-term use.

HRT use in breast cancer survivors

Women who have had breast cancer present their doctors with a dilemma. Several observational studies have suggested that there is no increased risk of breast cancer recurrence or death in women with breast cancer who are given HRT to relieve severe menopausal symptoms that cannot be treated otherwise. However, the follow-up periods in these studies were short and the women were likely to have early stage disease.[93]

A number of prospective trials are currently underway, but data will not be available for several years.

HRT and family history of breast cancer

Family history is an important risk factor for breast cancer, and there is often concern in prescribing HRT for postmenopausal women with a positive family history. In a further publication of the collaborative re-analysis, the issue of a potential impact of HRT on breast cancer in these women could not be addressed due to insufficient numbers of cases and controls using HRT for a sufficient length of time.[94] It is difficult to be sure that women with a family history of breast cancer do not have a different breast cancer risk on HRT from other women. However, their underlying risk is higher due to their family history.

Endometrial cancer

Effect of unopposed oestrogen therapy

Unopposed oestrogen therapy increases the risk of developing both endometrial hyperplasia and endometrial cancer in postmenopausal women with an intact uterus. In a Cochrane review, the odds of developing any type of endometrial hyperplasia were dependent on dose and duration of unopposed oestrogen therapy,[95] ranging from 5.4 to 16.0 in women taking "moderate" doses from 6 to 36 months duration of treatment. The meta-analysis clearly shows a dose-response and duration of treatment-response relationship between oestrogen use and risk of endometrial hyperplasia. The relative risk of endometrial cancer in women using oestrogen compared to non-users has been estimated as 2.3 (95% CI 2.1–2.5), with a much higher relative risk associated with prolonged duration of use (RR = 9.5 for 10 or more years). The relative risk of endometrial cancer remains elevated 5 or more years after discontinuation of oestrogen.

Effect of combined oestrogen and progestogen HRT

Most of the evidence for combined HRT is based on cohort and case-control studies – one meta-analysis reported that overall there was no increased risk of endometrial cancer in women taking combined HRT (RR=0.8, 95% CI 0.6–1.2).[96]

In the discontinued arm of the WHI study, endometrial cancer risk was similar for continuous combined treatment and the placebo group (HR 0.83, CI 0.47–1.47).[43]

Observational studies suggest that sequential regimens are less effective than continuous regimens. A recent large case-control study[97] indicated that endometrial cancer risk in combined HRT users was dependent on the duration of the progestogen dose. Sequential therapy, where progestogen was administered for more than 10 days per month, and continuous therapy did not increase risk of endometrial cancer. However, other case-control studies have found that sequential combined HRT, regardless of progestogen duration, is associated with an increased risk of endometrial cancer compared with non-users in long-term users.[98, 99]

Risk of endometrial hyperplasia

There is more conclusive evidence of the effects of combined therapy on the development of endometrial hyperplasia. In the Cochrane review,[95] the odds of developing hyperplasia were significantly reduced in the combined oestrogen-progestogen groups (both continuous and sequential regimens) when compared with the unopposed-oestrogen groups and there were no statistically significant differences in rates when combined therapy was compared with placebo groups.

Combined versus sequential regimens

Sequential regimens may be less effective than combined regimens in preventing endometrial cancer, and there is good evidence that continuous treatment is more effective in preventing hyperplasia.

In the PEPI trial,[23] only 0.8% of women receiving a continuous combined regimen of CEE (0.625 mg) plus MPA (2.5 mg) had hyperplasia after 3 years of treatment. However, a 5% incidence of endometrial hyperplasia was reported in groups where women received CEE (0.625 mg) plus cyclic MPA (10 mg) or CEE (0.625 mg) plus cyclic micronized progesterone (200 mg). In these groups, progestogens were given for 12 days of each cycle.

Another large randomized controlled trial of 1176 women reported that after 1 year, all doses of norethindrone acetate (0.1 mg, 0.25 mg, 0.5 mg) given continuously gave adequate endometrial protection when used with 1 mg oestradiol. At 12 months, the incidence of hyperplasia was 14.6% with unopposed oestradiol (1 mg) and 0.8%, 0.4% and 0.4% with 0.1 mg, 0.25 mg and 0.5 mg norethindrone acetate respectively.[100]

Duration of progestogen in sequential regimens
Sequential HRT therapy with progestogen (all types combined) administered for 12 days or more appears to be more effective than shorter courses of progestogen.[95] However, some studies do suggest that a regimen of 10 days of progestogen in sequential regimens offers adequate endometrial protection.

Other regimens
In "long cycle" HRT, a progestogen is given every 2, 3 or 4 months to lessen the impact of side-effects and improve adherence to therapy. However, a trial of long cycle HRT (progestogen given every 3 months for 10 days) versus standard HRT (progestogen given monthly for 10 days) in 240 women was discontinued after 3–4 years because of significantly higher hyperplastic changes in the long cycle HRT group.[101]

HRT after endometrial cancer

Endometrial cancer has traditionally been considered a contra-indication to HRT. Three observational retrospective studies have assessed the impact of oestrogen replacement after endometrial cancer.[102–104] In all three studies, lower rates of cancer recurrence and death were seen in the groups treated with oestrogen. A large multi-centre, randomized controlled trial in the US is currently recruiting women with previous stage 1 or 2 endometrial cancer since 1997 to compare daily CEE with placebo over 3 years. Until this trial reports, there is insufficient evidence on which to base recommendations.

Ovarian cancer

World-wide, ovarian cancer is the sixth most common cancer among women. In the US, the life-time risk for 50-year-old women of developing ovarian cancer is relatively low (1.7% compared to 11.9% for breast cancer and 2.8% for endometrial cancer), but most cases are diagnosed at an advanced stage and prognosis is poor.

The effect of HRT on risk is unclear. A systematic review of 11 case-control and cohort studies concluded that use of HRT for more than 10 years increased the risk of developing ovarian cancer,[105] findings confirmed by another meta-analysis of observational studies.[106] A recent large cohort study of 211,581 women followed over 14 years reported that postmenopausal oestrogen use for 10 or more years was associated with an increased risk of ovarian cancer mortality, which persisted up to 20 years after cessation of use.[107] Another US cohort study with 44,241 women and 329 incident cases suggested that women who use oestrogen-only therapy, particularly for 10 years or more, were at increased risk.[108] One systematic review of 15 case-control trials reported no association between the use of oestrogen replacement therapy and ovarian cancer risk.[109] However, one recent Swedish case-control study reported increased risk for use exceeding 10 years. Risk appeared largely confined to oestrogen plus sequential use of progestins, not continuous combined HRT.[110] To date, most of the studies have only considered women who have used unopposed medium potency oestrogens and there is little information on the role of combined HRT.

HRT after ovarian cancer

Treatment for ovarian cancer includes bilateral salpingo-oophorectomy that induces a premature menopause in premenopausal women. Premature menopause is associated with a greater likelihood of unpleasant menopausal symptoms and a long-term risk of osteoporosis.

A randomized controlled trial of 130 women with ovarian cancer followed for 4 years has confirmed that post-operative oestrogen replacement did not have a negative effect on either the disease-free interval or overall survival of ovarian cancer survivors.[111]

Cervical cancer

Observational studies do not suggest that cervical cancer should be regarded as a contra-indication to HRT.[112]

Colorectal cancer

In Western countries, deaths from colorectal cancer in postmenopausal women are close to those due to breast cancer.

Meta-analyses have reported that the risk of either colon or rectal cancer with ever use of HRT was not significantly reduced. [113, 114] However, a subgroup analysis based on seven studies, demonstrated a decreased risk of colorectal cancer with recent use of HRT within the last year (OR = 0.67, 95% CO 0.59–0.77).[113] With the exception of one case-control study, all observational data have shown that colorectal cancer is not increased with HRT. In the WHI trial, colorectal cancer risk was reduced in the group assigned to CEE 0.625 mg and MPA 2.5 mg daily. The hazard ratio was 0.63 (CI 0.43–0.92), reaching nominal significance.[43]

HRT and Risk of Venous Thromboembolism

HRT is associated with an increased risk of VTE. Observational studies have established that oestrogen replacement doubles the risk of VTE and pulmonary embolism. This increase in risk is seen with both oral and transdermal preparations. However, the increase in risk should be considered in the context of the population baseline risk in women aged 45–64 years, which is around one case per 10,000 women. Therefore, the absolute risk is low, at around three cases per 10,000 treated women per year.[115]

Pathophysiology

The pathophysiology of oestrogen-induced VTE is not well understood. It is thought that oestrogen has effects on vascular endothelium and on coagulation factors that may influence the potential for VTE. A recent double-blind study randomized women who had experienced VTE to HRT (continuous oestrogen and norethisterone acetate) or placebo for 2 years. HRT caused increases in markers of activated coagulation (prothrombin fragments 1+2, thrombin-antithrombin complex, and D-diner) after 3 months of treatment and reduced levels of the anticoagulants antithrombin and protein C by 12–17%. The increase in markers was greatest in those women who went on to have another VTE event, but was similar in carriers and non-carriers of the factor V Leiden mutation.[116]

A follow-up study of the PEPI trial found that women with VTE had lower baseline fibrinogen levels than women without VTE – although the clinical relevance of this is not clear.

Oestrogen replacement and the risk of VTE

A recent meta-analysis has assessed the risk for VTE. Twelve studies of oestrogen were identified: three randomized, eight case-control studies and one cohort study.[117] When the data were pooled, current oestrogen use was found to be associated with an increased risk of VTE (relative risk 2.14, 95% CI

1.64–2.81). The baseline risk was estimated at 1.3 per 10,000 woman-years and, therefore, the absolute rate increase was 1.5 VTE events per 10,000 women in 1 year (Figure 24).

Evidence from six case-control studies that reported risk according to duration of use found that the relative risk was highest in the first year of use (relative risk 3.49, 95% CI 2.33–5.59). The absolute incremental risk was 3.2 additional events for the first 12 months and 1.2 additional events after 12 months (Figure 25).

In the WHI trial, the hazard ratio was 2.11 (CI 1.58–2.82) for venous thromboembolic disease; 2.07 (CI 1.49–2.87) for deep vein thrombosis, and 2.13 (CI 1.3– 325) for pulmonary embolism.[43] No noteworthy interaction with age, smoking status, aspirin or statin use were found for the effect of oestrogen plus progestin.

Risk was higher in the studies that included women with coronary artery disease. It should be noted that the studies included in the meta-analysis had a number of important limitations:

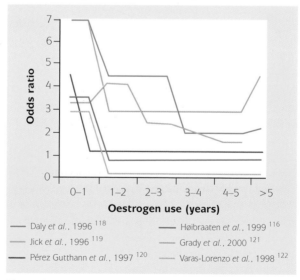

Figure 24. Odds ratio for thromboembolic events were higher in the first or second year than in subsequent years in all six studies reporting by year of us. Reproduced with permission from Annals of Internal Medicine, reference 117.

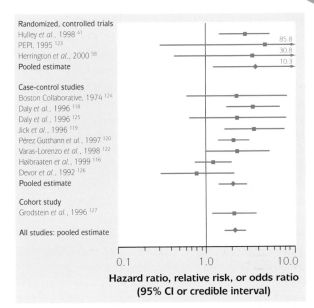

Figure 25. Meta-analysis of oestrogen studies. Reproduced with permission from Annals of Internal Medicine, reference 117.

- Methods for diagnosing VTE were inconsistent among studies, and, because accurate diagnosis of deep vein thrombosis is difficult, cases may have been misclassified, which could have affected study outcomes in either direction
- Eligibility criteria differed among studies – the observational studies tended to enrol younger, healthier women and excluded those with a history of coronary artery disease
- Race was not indicated in a number of studies – there is some evidence that there is an increased risk of VTE in African–American women

Patients at high risk of VTE

The HERS study[121] reported increased risk of VTE in patients with:

- Hip or lower extremity fractures

- Cancer
- Hospitalization
- Surgery
- Later onset of menopause (aged >52 years)

Other expected risk factors (hypertension, smoking and BMI) did not predict events. Statin use and aspirin were protective. Other studies have shown that women with a previous VTE and women with factor V Leiden mutation are also at higher risk.

VTE and raloxifene

The largest study of raloxifene, the MORE study,[128] found a three-fold increase in risk with daily raloxifene use over a 3-year period. This contrasts with smaller, earlier studies that did not see an increase in events.

HRT after VTE

The AACE guidelines for the Management of Menopause,[6] state that previous VTE is a relative contra-indication to HRT, but emphasize that the reality of the thrombotic event must be evaluated, and that around 50% of VTE is misdiagnosed.

The Royal College of Obstetricians and Gynaecologists has issued recommendations regarding HRT and VTE (Table 34).[12]

Recommendations from Royal College of Obstetricians and Gynaecologists regarding HRT and VTE
There is no indication for routine screening for thrombophilia in women starting HRT.
Women starting HRT should have a personal and family history taken of VTE events.
Women starting on HRT should have an assessment made of additional risk factors for thrombotic disease.
Women with a personal or family history of VTE should undergo a thrombophilia screen.

Table 34. Recommendations from Royal College of Obstetricians and Gynaecologists regarding HRT and VTE.

Future Developments

The mechanism of action of oestrogens is still not fully understood but major steps have been achieved in the last decade in the understanding of receptor-mediated effects. The discovery of a second oestrogen receptor and an interaction between oestrogen receptors and other steroid receptors, as well as the role of cytokines in modifying receptor responses, is now acknowledged. This research has led to an increased understanding as to why some substances, such as SERMs, can act as oestrogen antagonists in some tissues and oestrogen agonists in other tissues. With this knowledge it is possible to target the original molecular structure to create novel compounds with higher selectivity. These groups of substances, commonly referred to as selective steroid receptor modulators, could be developed to exert only desirable effects, thus avoiding the side-effects and also enhancing the desirable effects. Full cortisone effects without bone loss or moon face appearance is an exciting prospect. In addition, it is possible to slightly alter the chemical structure and, thereby, perhaps the pharmacokinetic and pharmacodynamic properties of steroid receptor modulators.

The drawbacks of long-term oestrogen replacement therapy have generated interest in developing alternatives to the traditional oestrogen treatment. Such alternatives comprise the use of naturally occurring compounds with oestrogenic properties, often referred to as phytoestrogens. Several such agents have been introduced on to the market, but existing products are too "weak" to be a real alternative to HRT for the treatment of hot flushes or diseases that postmenopausal women encounter.

However, many of the active substances have been identified and classified according to their chemical structure, and the so-called purified phytoestrogens are under development. About 100 plants, some of which are edible, contain a variety of at least 30 specific compounds in total, which are known to exhibit oestrogenic activity in humans and animals. Phytoestrogens consist of a number of classes: isoflavones, lignans, coumestans and fungal oestrogens. Various legumes contain the isoflavones daidzein, genistein, formononetin, biochanin A and the coumestan coumestrol.

It has become increasingly clear that the mandatory addition of progestogens to protect the endometrium from malignant transformations by oestrogen stimulation is not problem-free. Women may accept monthly bleeds around the menopause and during the following years, but, with advancing age, bleed-free regimens are clearly preferred.

This desired outcome can be achieved in a great many women by using continuous combined regimens, but some of the recipients of such therapy may bleed from an atrophic endometrium. Monitoring, surveillance and treatment of bleeds from an atrophic endometrium remains a challenge as we do not fully understand the aetiology underlying these atrophic bleeds, although much knowledge has been gained during the past few years.

The alleviation or even abolition of the problem of uterine bleeding using endometrial ablation by hysterectomy remains to be proven in well-designed studies with appropriate long-term follow-up. The recent WHI data augment interest in safe oestrogen monotherapy and hence also in pharmacotherapy and devices rendering progestogen addition unnecessary.

To induce endometrial atrophy, and thereby a bleed-free regimen, the progestogen influence needs to be fairly high. This means that other progestogenic side-effects are not uncommon in women using continuous combined regimens. Therefore, we need to use more selective progestogens primarily designed as oestrogen co-medications for the elderly postmenopausal woman. Unfortunately, it is still the case that almost all data on the pharmocokinetics and pharmacodynamics of oestrogens, progestogens and various oestrogen/progestogen combinations (including the continuous combined regimens) are obtained from women around 50 years of age, and such data are probably not transferable to an older population. For these reasons, we have insufficient data to guide us to select progestogen type, dose or mode of administration in late postmenopausal women.

Cost-benefit analyses seem to suggest that oestrogens are cost effective in women with symptoms and particularly in women without a uterus. This implies that the only proven positive effect of progestogen is its reduction of endometrial hyperplasia and endometrial cancer. Thus, oestrogens can be given to the hysterectomized woman without progestogen co-medication. However, this should not encourage the medical community to perform hysterectomies around the time of the menopause.

Development of oestrogen components

The predominant human natural oestrogen during the fertile period is 17β-oestradiol. Hence, several therapies focus on the use of oestradiol. Many of the same problems of natural progesterone also arise with natural oestradiol. We need to know what molecular substituents are responsible for the positive effects on symptoms and prevention, and what molecular substituents may contribute to weight gain and influence breast tissues, i.e. the proliferation of glandular cells. Proliferation of these cells is thought to be involved in the development of breast cancer. The oestradiol molecule could be "tailored", in particular to diminish or even abolish the interaction with breast tissues.

Another feature to look at is the various components of conjugated equine oestrogens. Although the main components are oestrone and oestrone sulphate, there are a variety of compounds that display different oestrogenic activities, and a few compounds appear to exert progestogenic and androgenic activities. In particular, the so-called alpha oestrogens, contained in conjugated equine oestrogens, are of interest as they possess qualities different from those of the beta compounds.

The further characterization of the various components of conjugated oestrogens and their biological effects should stimulate future research into oestrogen pharmacology and pharmacodynamics. It is also of extreme importance to try to identify the type of molecular infrastructure that is responsible for the various cardiovascular effects, such as antioxidative properties and vasodilatation, as well as the bone sparing effects. However, one may wonder whether non-human, though natural, oestrogens are the best possible treatment option today given the availabilty of 17β-oestradiol.

New delivery systems have been introduced to improve the convenience of treatment and the potential for long-term use. A vaginal silicone ring with a release of 7.5 μg oestradiol per day constantly over a period of 3 months seems to be a valuable addition in the treatment of urogenital symptoms in oestrogen-deprived women. Vaginal tablets containing 25 μg estradiol to be applied twice weekly are other alternatives to vaginal creams containing oestriol or conjugated oestrogens. Hormone-containing patches and gels are now established but these need improvement to avoid local skin irritation. The recently introduced nasal spray continues to be an interesting line of development. Other forms of local treatment, though systemic absorption seems to be possible, include oestradiol eye drops designed to help symptoms such as dry eye.

Long-acting delivery systems, such as oestradiol implants and intramuscular injection, have been used for many years in various European countries. However, supraphysiological blood levels are commonly seen associated with the phenomenon of symptom recurrence and tachyphylaxis. Non-biodegradable silicone-based implants could provide an improvement for this type of replacement to avoid peak levels after insertion and maintain lower, more constant oestradiol levels in the range of that found in the early to mid-follicular phase.

An additional intriguing approach is the external regulation of intrabodily hormone containing devices. This can be achieved by the so-called blue tooth technique, which is under development in co-operation with the telecom industry. Many medical problems could benefit immensely from such techniques, including insulin administration in diabetics but also sex steroids and anticoagulant therapy.

Long-cycle therapy addresses a major problem, uterine bleeding, which is not accepted by most women. Although it is a very intriguing idea to space out the sequential administration of a progestogen to induce endometrial shedding, it should be noted that the long-term endometrial safety of the few combinations tested remains to be demonstrated.

Development of progestogens and progesterone

An important task for future research is to try to delineate which structures in the progesterone molecule yield the different metabolic aspects. In other words, what molecular structures influence the endometrium and what molecular specifications give other potential negative effects, such as PMS-like effects and lowering of HDL cholesterol. So far, progestogens have been developed mostly as constituents in contraceptives and to treat various bleeding disorders. However, more recently, progestogens have become an important feature in newer agents for postmenopausal women.

The development of newer progestogens with fewer side-effects and a more selective influence on the endometrium is an obvious goal in this respect. The patch administration of oestrogens is favoured; however, progestogens cannot be administered via the transdermal route as some of them have very little or no first pass hepatic metabolism, as demonstrated by levonorgestrel. Other progestogens, including progesterone, may show a significant first pass metabolism.

Natural progesterone displays a low oral bioavailability. Using newer micro-crystalization techniques it has been possible to achieve an acceptable bioavailability via the oral route. However, this needs to be substantially improved as only a small fraction of orally administered progesterone is bioavailable. This means that progesterone has to be given in doses of 200 mg per day to ensure endometrial protection. Work is underway to modify the molecule so that it may be absorbed either via the skin or the oral route and is then rapidly degraded to natural progesterone. It is disputable which type of progestogen one should prefer, i.e. one that has similar pharmacokinetics to the administered oestrogens, such as MPA, norethisterone or dydrogesterone, or a more long-acting progestogen, such as desogestrel, levonorgestrel or norgestimate.

A vaginal progesterone gel that is administered twice weekly for a period of 1 month at a dose of 45 mg has been shown to induce a secretory endometrium in the presence of mean serum progesterone levels as low as 2 ng/ml. This is suggestive of a so-called first uterine pass effect in women with premature ovarian failure and ovarian dysgenesis.[130] Endometrial safety remains to be demonstrated in clinical long-term trials of postmenopausal women. Other developments to improve acceptance by women without compromising endometrial safety are to administer or use various progestogens as implants or intrauterine devices. One approved intrauterine device releases levonorgestrel 20 µg daily for 5 years.

Two different intrauterine devices with a release rate of 5 and 10 µg/24 h were reported to induce acceptable bleeding patterns and showed beneficial effects on lipid and lipoprotein metabolism when combined with 2 mg oestradiol valerate that was orally administered. A disadvantage with this type of device is that the progestogen reservoir covered by the rate-limiting membrane could be too thick for insertion into the uterus of a postmenopausal woman. A device with a thinner vertical arm needs to be developed should the use be extended to postmenopausal women. A release rate of 5–10 µg/24 h is sufficient for endometrial protection.

Another feature is to introduce newer regimens to reduce the progestogen dosage. An example of this is the so called "on-and-off therapy" in which oestrogens are given continuously and progestogens are given 3 days on and 3 days off. In such clinical trials, bleeding discomforts was acceptable; however, both extensive clinical experience and well-designed studies are lacking.

It may be an intriguing concept to use oestrogens as adjunct therapy to other (chronic) medications, such as insulin or thyroid hormones. Indeed some data indicate that an additive effect by oestrogens seems plausible with bisphosphonates for osteoporosis prevention. Currently combinations of oestrogens and a variety of antihypertensive drugs to delineate perceived additive or even synergistic effects are under investigation. This is particularly prudent because oestrogen is about the only compound that has a great effect, albeit small, on diastolic rather than systolic blood pressure. An ACE-inhibiting effect and calcium channel blocking effect have been demonstrated for oestrogens, and research combining oestrogens with different classes of anti hypertensive drugs could improve the overall effect and possibly also decrease untoward side-effects by several of the compounds involved.

In conclusion, it is a challenge to define those women who have the most to gain from the administration of oestrogens (and progestogens when necessary) in order to make it truly beneficial and cost-effective.

Last, but not least, it should be pointed out that women should of course be counselled that HRT is only one option provided by the medical community. The other options should include evidence-based advice about the best possible life style including nutrition, weight control, and physical exercise in order to prevent disease.

Frequently Asked Questions

Why do not all women have hot flushes?

Unfortunately there is no definitive answer to this question as we do not fully understand the exact nature of the hot flush. But we do know the following. The severity of flushes is coupled to the change per time unit (and not the absolute levels) of hormones, especially oestrogens. Therefore women who undergo ovariectomy are often hit hard. In women in whom oestrogen levels decline slowly, e.g. in obesity, symptoms are often less severe. There is also a genetic disposition, so a woman's symptomatology is likely to be similar to her mother's.

Why do men not have climacteric symptoms?

This is a common misconception. Men do get climacteric symptoms but only under special circumstances, such as orchidectomy or heavy cytostatic treatment. This will result in an instant cessation of testosterone secretion leading to a similar symptomatology as occurs in women. Whether this is due to the decline in testosterone or the concomitant rapid decline in brain tissue oestradiol remains to be clarified. There appears to be circumstantial evidence that some men without these conditions may also have hot flushes. However, there are no good studies that have looked into this matter more systematically.

Are laboratory tests useful to establish menopause?

In some cases, such as in hysterectomized women, the measurement of FSH may be helpful. High levels (>30 IU indicate menopause. Other endocrine diseases, especially in women at ages around 40–45 years, may be the explanatory mechanism behind symptoms such as flushes. The huge inter- and intraindividual variation of oestradiol renders the measurement of this hormone less reliable as a diagnostic tool.

Will menopause impact negatively on my sex life?

Not necessarily. In fact, it may even improve as the fear of pregnancy is no longer present. Sometimes dyspareunia (due to low grade lubrication) may occur, which can be easily treated with (topical) oestrogen administration. Sometimes lubricants without oestrogen may also offer some help.

When can I stop thinking about contraception?

Fertility declines gradually from the age of 35. After age 45 pregnancies are rare, particularly in women with an irregular bleeding pattern and/or climacteric symptoms. In women with regular cycles ovulations do occur and, albeit rare, the possibility of pregnancy cannot be totally negated until cessation of menses. For women above the age of 40–45 years it may be helpful to discuss which option is best for contraception as there are a variety of possibilities, including intrauterine devices, barrier methods (condoms), and oral contraceptives (some of which may only contain progestogen-only pills).

Will menopause make my skin more sensitive to the sun?

With advancing age the skin becomes thinner with less blood circulation. This process is further enhanced by oestrogen deficiency. But as skin sensitivity is more a function of age, treatment with HRT may not restore total skin health. The risk of skin cancers also increase with age, irrespective of hormonal influence. Therefore, a prudent sun protection is recommended. Please note that smoking is also bad for the skin.

Will I lose my breast size when I enter menopause?

The most abundant component of the female breast is fat. The fatty content of the mammary gland declines as a function of the aging process and oestrogen deficiency. To some extent (but not entirely) this may be counteracted by oestrogen treatment.

How long should I continue taking HRT?

So long as you have climacteric symptoms. It is a good idea to assess whether you need HRT once a year, particularly after 4–5 years. You may also wish to decrease the oestrogen dose gradually as time goes by. There is no need to interrupt treatment with vaginal oestrogen preparations unless you wish to do so.

Will my symptoms relapse after HRT?

There is a good chance that symptoms will gradually decline once you stop HRT. Some women do not experience any symptoms once HRT is stopped. Unfortunately, we do not know why women react so differently.

How do I know if I have menopausal symptoms if I am using oral contraceptives or HRT?

It may be that you do not have climacteric symptoms because you take hormonal contraception. It may be a good idea to observe yourself to see whether you have hot flushes in the pill-free interval. If so, this could be an indication that you no longer need contraception.

It is only when you stop taking HRT that you will be able to see whether you have hot flushes or sweats again or whether your sleep is disrupted.

Will I get breast cancer if I take HRT?

Breast cancer is a common disease and it can occur in women regardless of whether they take oral contraceptives or HRT. Please discuss with your doctor whether you should continue to take HRT after 4–5 years. There are studies suggesting that long-term HRT increases the relative risk of breast cancer.

Are there any other risks or benefits with HRT?

HRT may help prevent fragility fractures (hip, spine) if taken for many years. Some studies suggest that colorectal cancers are found less often in women who take HRT. Some women find their memory is better with HRT. Sleeping problems that developed at the time of the menopausal transition may be helped with HRT. The same holds true for depressive symptoms. But keep in mind that depression diagnosed before the menopause is by and large not a reason to start HRT.

Are there alternatives for prevention of osteoporosis?
Yes, there are. You may wish to discuss alternative treatments with your doctor. It is important to rethink your diet and your level of physical activity. Calcium and vitamin D are both essential for your bones throughout life and you should ensure that you eat plenty of calcium-rich foods, such as milk products, certain vegetables (broccoli) and vitamin-D rich foods (sea fish).

What should I do if I gain weight when taking HRT?
Please look at you diet and your level of physical activity. It is a fact that most people, women and men, gain weight after age 30. Try to establish a personal scheme with regular exercise and healthy nutrition, cut back on unsaturated fats and eat more (green) vegetables and fresh fruits. Try to use the lowest possible dose of oestrogen anyway, regardless of whether you have a weight problem.

Does HRT prevent Alzheimer's disease?
Studies looking at women who chose HRT many years ago indicate that HRT can prevent the onset of Alzheimer's disease. However, there are no large clinical trials available to give us much-needed information as to whether oestrogen helps maintain brain function into old age.

Does HRT prevent incontinence?
Some women do find oestrogens helpful when a certain type of incontinence prevails, such as stress incontinence. There are no good studies to show that HRT is indeed effective. Again, special physical exercises are helpful, as are some specific medications and special surgical procedures.

Do I need to have more gynaecological examinations, mammography and other laboratory tests once I start taking HRT?
No. Please keep to your regular routine of carrying out regular breast exams, as well as having mammograms and smears to

detect cervical cancer. There is no need to check blood levels of hormones once you take HRT. The best way to check whether your HRT regimen is good for you is to watch, yourself, whether your symptoms are gone.

Can I take HRT if I have a uterine fibroid?

Yes; it is possible that you may experience irregular bleeding at the beginning of therapy.

I have diabetes. May I take HRT?

Yes, you can take HRT to counteract your climacteric symptoms. Check with your doctor to make sure that you use the lowest dose possible to help your symptoms. For vaginal problems use topical treatments. Make sure that your diabetes treatment (medication, diet) is optimal.

I had a MI. Can HRT help prevent further heart disease?

Please see your doctor to get the best possible advice as to whether you should use specific drugs to help your cardiovascular system. We do not have good data to show that oestrogens are helpful to prevent further heart disease.

Are there other ways apart from HRT to alleviate hot flushes?

Sometimes flushes can be alleviated if you avoid spicy food, alcoholic beverages, coffee or black tea. Some plants may also be helpful, such as extracts from black kohosh. However, there are no long-term studies to show what plant extracts do. The same holds true for medications and food supplements called phytoestrogens.

Does HRT help with wrinkles or loss of hair?

As women and men grow older this is a problem that many of us encounter. You should take good care of your skin, stop smoking (if you smoke) and make sure that your diet contains enough vitamins and minerals. There are no good studies to show that HRT prevents wrinkles or stops hair loss. However, in some women, hair loss may be associated with high androgen levels, so in this special situation HRT may be of some help.

Is it good or bad to have bleedings once I use HRT?
Some HRT regimens produce bleeding and some do not. It is up to you to choose which you prefer.

My mother had a deep vein thrombosis after she started HRT. Could this also happen to me?
As women and men grow older the risk of deep vein thrombosis increases. The risk also increases with obesity. Without HRT, 1–2 women in 10,000 will get a thrombosis each year. Oestrogens appear to affect an extra 2–3 women in 10,000 per year. This is only an estimate. The risk is largely confined to the first year of treatment. There is a possibility that your personal risk is larger because of your genetic predisposition. Please ask your doctor whether you should have a special laboratory test.

I have already osteoporosis and I sustained a vertebral fracture. Should I start HRT to prevent further bone loss ?
Oestrogens may slow down bone loss. However, there are no convincing studies to suggest that the future risk of a further vertebral fracture, or any other fracture (hip, wrist) is diminished. Please ask your doctor whether you should start treatment with a bisphosphonate or raloxifene. It is also important to check your diet. Make sure your daily calcium intake is within the range of 1000–1500 mg and vitamin D in the range of 800 IU per day.

I am 70 and have still flushes. Is this normal? Can I take oestrogens?
Some women continue to have flushes well beyond the age of 50. We do not know why. There are other very rare conditions that may be linked to flushes, such as diabetes, thyroid disease and tumours of the adrenal gland. Low doses

of oestrogens may help alleviate flushes. However, the risk of thrombosis, although very small, is greater compared to women in their fifties.

I have had breast cancer /endometrial cancer. I cannot tolerate my flushes anymore, so can I take oestrogens?

Oestrogens will help with the climacteric symptoms. However, make sure that this treatment does not negatively interfere with your cancer treatment. Studies looking at women who decided to use oestrogens suggest that oestrogens do not negatively affect the further development of the underlying disease once breast (or endometrial cancer) has been treated.

I have migraines, can I take HRT?

Some women have less migraines with HRT, whereas other women have more. If you are considering taking HRT, please discuss with your doctor to ascertain which type of headache or migraine you have. It may be helpful to remember whether taking oral contraceptives had any effect on your headaches or migraines.

Does my partner also need HRT?

Men do not have a menopause. However, there are various hormonal systems that change with age. There are no studies at present to suggest that men should take hormones (androgens, testosterone or female hormones, such as oestrogens) to prevent disease.

References

1. Abernethy K. *The Menopause and HRT*. 2nd edition. Bailliere Tindall, 2001.

2. Anasti JN. Premature ovarian failure: an update. *Fertil Steril* 1998; **70**: 1–15.

3. Devi A, Benn PA. X chromosome abnormalities in women with premature ovarian failure. *J Reprod Med* 1999; **4**: 321–324.

4. Seely T, Ashton S. Premature ovarian failure: a practical approach. *J Br Menopause Soc* 2000; **6**: 107–109.

5. Howell SJ, Berger G , Adams JE *et al*. Bone mineral density in women with cytotoxic ovarian failure. *Clin Endocrinol* 1998; **49**: 397–402.

6. AACE medical guidelines for clinical practice for management of menopause. *Endocr Pract* 1999; **5**: 355–366.

7. Ratner S, Ofri D. Menopause and hormone replacement: Part 1. Evaluation and treatment. *West J Med* 2001; **174**: 400–404.

8. McKinlay SM, Brambilla PJ, Posner JG. The normal menopause transition. *Maturitas* 1992; **14**: 103–115.

9. Greendale GA, Lee NP, Arriola ER. The menopause. *Lancet* 1999; **353**: 571–580.

10. Greendale GA, Reboussin BA, Hogan P *et al*. Symptom relief and side effects of postmenopausal hormones: results from the Postmenopausal Estrogen/Progestin Interventions Trial. *Obstet Gynecol* 1998; **92**: 982–988.

11. Nagamani M, Kelver ME, Smith ER. Treatment of menopausal hot flashes with transdermal administration of clonidine. *Am J Obstet Gynecol* 1987; **156**: 561–565.

12. Loprinzi CL, Michalak JC, Quella SK *et al*. Megestrol acetate for the prevention of hot flashes. *N Engl J Med* 1994; **331**: 347–352.

13. Ishiko O, Hirai K, Sumi T *et al*. Hormone replacement therapy plus pelvic floor muscle exercise for postmenopausal

stress incontinence. A randomized, controlled trial. *J Reprod Med* 2001; **46**: 213–220.

14. Fantl JA, Cardozo L, McClish DK. Estrogen therapy in the management of urinary incontinence in post-menopausal women: a meta–analysis. *Obstet Gynecol* 1994; **83**: 12–18.

15. Grady D, Brown JS, Vittinghoff E *et al.* for The HERS Research Group. Postmenopausal hormones and incontinence: the Heart and Estrogen/Progestin Replacement Study. *Obstet Gynecol* 2001; **97**: 116–120.

16. Raz R, Stamm WE. A controlled trial of intravaginal estriol in postmenopausal women with recurrent urinary tract infections. *N Engl J Med* 1993; **329**: 753–759.

17. Bygdeman M, Swahn ML. Replens versus dienoestrol cream in the symptomatic treatment of vaginal atrophy in postmenopausal women. *Maturitas* 1996; **23**: 259–263.

18. Dennerstein L, Randolph J, Taffe J *et al*. Hormones, mood, sexuality, and the menopausal transition. *Fertil Steril* 2002; **77** (Suppl 4): 42–48.

19. Shifren L, Braunstein GD, Simon JA *et al*. Transdermal testosterone treatment in postmenopausal women with impaired sexual function after oophorectomy. *N Engl J Med* 2000; **343**: 682–688.

20. Strickler R, Stovall DW, Merritt D *et al*. Raloxifene and estrogen effects on quality of life in healthy postmenopausal women: a placebo-controlled randomized trial. *Obstet Gynecol* 2000; **96**: 359–365.

21. Andersson K, Mattsson LA, Milsom I. Use of hormone replacement therapy. *Lancet* 1996; **348**: 1521.

22. Rubin GL, Peterson HB, Lee NC *et al*. Estrogen replacement therapy and the risk of endometrial cancer: remaining controversies. *Am J Obstet Gynecol* 1990; **162**: 148–154.

23. The Writing Group for the PEPI Trial: Effects of hormonal replacement therapy on endometrial histology in postmenopausal women. *JAMA* 1996; **275**: 370–375.

24. Hänggi W, Lippuner K, Riesen W *et al*. Long-term influence of different postmenopausal hormone replacement

regimen on serum lipids and lipoprotein(a). A randomized study. *Br J Obstet Gynaecol* 1997; **104**: 708–717.

25. Bachman G, Bancroft J, Braunstein G *et al*. Female androgen insufficiency: the Princeton consensus statement on definition, classification, and assessment. *Fertil Steril* 2002; 660–665.

26. Kaplan HS, Owett T. The female androgen deficiency syndrome. *J Sex Marital Ther* 1993; **19**: 3–24.

27. Cardozo L, Gibb DM, Tuck SM *et al*. The effects of subcutaneous hormone implants during climacteric. *Maturitas* 1984; **5**: 177–184.

28. Burger HG, Hailes J, Menelaus M *et al*. The management of persistent menopausal symptoms with oestradiol-testosterone implants: Clinical, lipid and hormonal results. *Maturitas* 1984; **6**: 351–358.

29. Sherwin BB, Gelfand MM, Brender W. Androgen enhances sexual motivation in females: A prospective, crossover study of sex steroid administration in the surgical menopause. *Psychosom Med* 1985; **47**: 339–351.

30. Sherwin BB, Gelfand MM. Differential symptom response to parenteral estrogen and/or androgen administration in the surgical menopause. *Am J Obstet Gynecol* 1985; **151**: 153–160.

31. Shifren JL, Braunstein GD, Casson PR *et al*. Transdermal testosterone treatment in women with impaired sexual function after oophorectomy. *N Engl J Med* 2000; **343**: 682–688.

32. Sarrel P, Dobay B, Wiita B. Estrogen and estrogen–androgen replacement in postmenopausal women dissatisfied with estrogen-only therapy. Sexual behavior and neuroendocrine responses. *J Reprod Med* 1998; **43**: 847–856.

33. Davis SR, McCloud PI, Strauss BJG *et al*. Testosterone enhances estradiol's effects on postmenopausal bone density and sexuality. *Maturitas* 1995; **21**: 227–236.

34. Compston JE. Sex steroids and bone. *Physiol Rev* 2001; **81**: 419–447.

35. Kanis JA, Melton LJ, Christiansen C *et al*. Perspective: The diagnosis of osteoporosis. *J Bone Miner Res* 1994; **9**: 1137–1141.

36. Cummings SR, Melton LJ. Epidemiology and outcomes of osteoporotic fractures. *Lancet* 2002; **359**; 1761–1767.

37. Reid IR, Chin K, Evans MC *et al*. Relation between increase of hip axis in older women in 1950s and 1990s and increase in age specific rates of hip fracture. *BMJ* 1994; **309**: 508–509.

38. Marcus R, Wong M, Heath H III *et al*. Antiresorptive treatment of postmenopausal osteoporosis; comparison of study designs and outcomes in large clinical trials with fracture as an endpoint. *Endocr Rev* 2002; **23**: 16–37.

39. Lufkin EG, Wahner HW, O'Fallon WM *et al*. Treatment of postmenopausal osteoporosis with transdermal oestrogen. *Ann Intern Med* 1992; **117**: 1–9.

40. Lindsay RD, Hart DM, Forrest C *et al*. Prevention of spinal osteoporosis in oophorectomised women. *Lancet* 1980; **2**: 1151–1154.

41. Hulley S, Grady D, Bush T *et al*. Randomized trial of estrogen plus progestin for secondary prevention of coronary heart disease in postmenopausal women. *JAMA* 1998; **280**: 605–613.

42. Komulainen M, Kroger H, Tuppurainen MT *et al*. Prevention of femoral and lumbar bone loss with hormone replacement therapy and vitamin D, in early postmenopausal women: A population–based 5–year randomized trial. *J Clin Endocrinol Metab* 1999; **84**: 546–552.

43. Writing Group for the Women´s Health Initiative Investigators. Risks and benefits of estrogen plus progestin in healthy postmenopausal women. *JAMA* 2002; **288**: 321–333.

44. Torgerson DJ, Bell-Syer SEM. Hormone replacement therapy and prevention of nonvertebral fractures. *JAMA* 2001; **285**: 2891–2897.

45. Jensen GF, Christiansen C, Transbol I. Treatment of post menopausal osteoporosis. A controlled therapeutic trial

comparing estrogen/gestagen, 1,25-dihydroxy-vitamin D3 and calcium. *Clin Endocrinol* 1982; **16**: 515–524.

46. Lufkin EG, Riggs BL.Three-year follow-up on effects of transdermal estrogen. *Ann Intern Med* 1996; **125**: 177.

47. Recker RR, Davies KM, Dowd RM *et al*. The effect of low-dose continuous estrogen and progesterone therapy with calcium and vitamin D on bone in elderly women –-A randomized, controlled trial. *Ann Intern Med* 1999; **130**: 897–904.

48. Felson DT, Zhang Y, Hannan MT *et al*. The effect of postmenopausal estrogen therapy on bone density in elderly women. *N Engl J Med* 1993; **329**: 1141–1146.

49. Ensrud KE, Palermo L, Black DM *et al*. Hip and calcaneal bone loss increase with advancing age: longitudinal results from the Study of Osteoporotic Fractures. *J Bone Miner Res* 1995; **10**: 1778–1787.

50. Schneider DL, Barrett-Connor EL, Morton DJ. Timing of postmenopausal estrogen for optimal bone mineral density — the Rancho Bernardo study. *JAMA* 1997; **277**: 543–547.

51. Greendale GA, Espeland M, Slone S *et al*. Bone mass response to discontinuation of long-term hormone replacement therapy: results from the postmenopausal estrogen/progestin (PEPI) safety follow–up study. *Arch Intern Med* 2002; **162**: 665–672.

52. Delmas PD. Treatment of postmenopausal osteoporosis. *Lancet* 2002; **359**: 2018–2026.

53. Ettinger B, Black DM, Mitlak BH *et al*. Reduction of vertebral fracture risk in postmenopausal women with osteoporosis treated with raloxifene – Results from a 3-year randomized clinical trial. *JAMA* 1999; **282**: 637–645.

54. Henderson BE, Paganini-Hill A, Ross RK. Decreased mortality in uses of estrogen replacement therapy. *Arch Intern Med* 1991; 75–78.

55. Ettinger B, Friedman GD, Bush T *et al*. Reduced mortality associated with long-term postmenopausal estrogen therapy. *Obstet Gynecol* 1996; **87**: 6–12.

56. Grodstein F, Stampfer MJ, Colditz GA *et al.*
Postmenopausal hormone therapy and mortality. *N Engl J Med*
1997; **336**: 1769–1775.

57. Stampfer MJ, Colditz GA. Estrogen replacement therapy
and coronary heart disease: a quantitative assessment of the
epidemiologic evidence. *Prev Med* 1991; **20**: 47–63.

58. Herrington DM, Reboussin DM, Brosnihan KB *et al.*
Effects of estrogen replacement on the progression of
coronary-artery atherosclerosis. *N Engl J Med* 2000; **343**:
522–529.

59. Clarke SC, Kelleher J, LLoyd-Jones H *et al.* A study of
hormone replacement therapy in postmenopausal women with
ischemic heart disease: The Papworth HRT Atherosclerosis
Study. *Br J Obstet Gynaecol* 2002; **109**: 1056–62.

60. Blumenthal RS, Zacur HA, Reis SE *et al.* Beyond the null
hypothesis — do the HERS results disprove the
estrogen/coronary heart disease hypothesis? *Am J Cardiol*
2000; **85**: 1015–1017.

61. Herrington DM, Vittinghoff E, Lin F *et al.* Statin therapy,
cardiovascular events, and total mortality on the Heart and
Estrogen/Progestin Replacement Study (HERS). *Circulation*
2002; **105**: 2962–2967.

62. Furberg CD, Vittinghoff E, Davidson M *et al.* Subgroup
interactions in the Heart and estrogen/progestin replacement
study. *Circulation* 2002; **105**: 917–922.

63. Grady D, Herrington D, Bittner V *et al.* for the HERS
Research Group. Cardiovascular disease outcomes during
6.8 years of hormone therapy: Heart and Estrogen/progestin
Replacement Study follow-up (HERS II). *JAMA* 2002; **288**:
49–57.

64. Mosca L, Collins P, Herrington DM *et al.* Hormone
replacement therapy and cardiovascular disease: a statement
for healthcare professionals from the American Heart
Association. *Circulation* 2001; **104**: 499–503.

65. Alexander KP, Newby LK, Hellkamp AS *et al.* Initiation of
hormone replacement therapy after acute myocardial
infarction is associated with more cardiac events during
follow-up. *J Am Coll Cardiol* 2001; **38**: 1–7.

66. Grodstein F, Manson JE, Stampfer MJ. Postmenopausal hormone use and secondary prevention of coronary events in the nurses' health study. A prospective, observational study. *Ann Intern Med* 2001; **135**: 1–8.

67. Barrett-Connor E, Grady D, Sashegyi A *et al*. Raloxifene and cardiovascular events in osteoporotic postmenopausal women: four-year results from the MORE (Multiple Outcomes of Raloxifene Evaluation) randomized trial. *JAMA* 2002; **287**: 847–857.

68. Grodstein F, Manson JE, Colditz GA *et al*. A prospective, observational study of postmenopausal hormone therapy and primary prevention of cardiovascular disease. *Ann Intern Med* 2000; **133**: 933–941.

69. Neves-e-Castro M, Samsioe G, Dören M, Skouby SO. Results from WHI and HERS II: Implications for women and the prescriber of HRT. *Maturitas* 2002; **42**: 255–8

70. Paganini-Hill A, Henderson VW. Estrogen deficiency and risk of Alzheimer's disease in women. *Am J Epidemiol* 1994; **140**: 256–261.

71. LeBlanc ES, Janowsky J, Chan BKS *et al*. Hormone replacement therapy and cognition. Systematic review and meta-analysis. *JAMA* 2001; **285**: 1489–1499.

72. Polo Kantola P, Portin R, Polo O *et al*. The effect of short-term estrogen replacement therapy on cognition: A randomized double-blind, cross-over trial in postmenopausal women. *Obstet Gynecol* 1998; **91**: 459–466.

73. Shaywitz SE, Shaywitz BA, Pugh KR *et al*. Effect of estrogen on brain activation patterns in postmenopausal women during working memory tasks. *JAMA* 1999; **281**: 1197–1202.

74. Hlatky MA, Boothroyd D, Vittinghoff E *et al*. Quality-of-life and depressive symptoms in postmenopausal women after receiving hormone therapy: results from the Heart and Estrogen/progestin Replacement Study (HERS). *JAMA* 2002; **28**: 591–597.

75. Yaffe K, Sawaya G, Lieberburg I *et al*. Estrogen therapy in postmenopausal women. *JAMA* 1998; **279**: 688–695.

76. Mulnard RA, Cotman CW, Kawas C *et al*. Estrogen replacement therapy for treatment of mild to moderate Alzheimer disease. *JAMA* 2000; **283**: 1007–1015.

77. Henderson VW, Paganini-Hill A, Miller BL *et al*. Estrogen for Alzheimer 's disease in women: Randomized, double-blind, placebo-controlled trial. *Neurology* 2000; **54**: 295–301.

78. Collaborative Group on Hormonal Factors in Breast Cancer. Breast cancer and hormone replacement therapy — collaborative reanalysis of data from 51 epidemiological studies of 52,705 women with breast cancer and 108,411 women without breast cancer. *Lancet* 1997; **350**: 1047–1059.

79. Gapstur SM, Morrow M, Sellers TA. Hormone replacement therapy and risk of breast cancer with favorable histology. Results of the Iowa Women's Health Study. *JAMA* 1999; **281**: 2091–2097.

80. Lando JF, Heck KE, Brett KM. Hormone replacement and breast cancer risk in a nationally representative cohort. *Am J Prev Med* 1999; **17**: 176–180.

81. Olsson H, Bladström A, Ingvar C *et al*. A population-based cohort study of HRT use and breast cancer in southern Sweden. *Br J Cancer* 2001; **85**: 674–677.

82. Smith–Warner SA, Spiegelman D, Yaun SS *et al*. Alcohol and breast cancer in women: A pooled analysis of cohort studies. *JAMA* 1998; **279**: 535–540.

83. Dupont WD, Page DL. Menopausal estrogen replacement therapy and breast cancer. *Arch Intern Med* 1991; **151**: 67–72.

84. Colditz GA, Hankinson SE, Hunter DJ. The use of estrogens and progestins and the risk of breast cancer in postmenopausal women. *N Engl J Med* 1995; **332**: 1589–1593.

85. Schairer C, Lubin J, Troisi R *et al*. Menopausal estrogen and estrogen-progestin replacement therapy and breast cancer risk. *JAMA* 2000; **283**: 485–491.

86. Persson I, Weiderpass E, Bergkvist L *et al*. Risks of breast and endometrial cancer after estrogen and estrogen-progestin replacement. *Cancer Causes Control* 1999; **10**: 253–260.

87. Magnusson C, Baron JA, Correia N *et al*. Breast–cancer risk following long-term oestrogen — and oestrogen-progestin replacement therapy. *Int J Cancer* 1999; **81**: 339–344.

88. Newcomb PA, Titus-Ernsthoff L, Egan KM *et al*. Postmenopausal estrogen and progestin use in relation to breast cancer risk. *Cancer Epidemiol Biomark Prev* 2002; **11**: 593–600

89. Kirsh V, Kreiger N. Estrogen and estrogen-progestin replacement therapy and risk of postmenopausal breast cancer in Canada. *Cancer Causes Control* 2002; **13**: 583–590

90. Chen C-L, Weiss NS, Newcomb P *et al*. Hormone replacement therapy in relation to breast cancer. *JAMA* 2002; **287**: 734–741

91. Nanda K, Bastian LA, Schulz K. Hormone replacement therapy and the risk of death from breast cancer: a systematic review. *Am J Obstet Gynecol* 2002; **186**: 325–334

92. Rodriguez C, Calle EE, Patel AV *et al*. Effect of body mass on the association between estrogen replacement therapy and mortality among elderly US women. *Am J Epidemiol* 2001; **153**: 145–152.

93. Col NF, Hirota LK, Orr RK *et al*. Hormone replacement therapy after breast cancer: a systematic review and quantitative assessment of risk. *J Clin Oncol* 2001; **19**: 2357–2363.

94. Collaborative Group on Hormonal Factors in Breast Cancer. Familial breast cancer: collaborative reanalysis of individual data from 52 epidemiological studies including 58 209 women with breast cancer and 101 986 women without the disease. *Lancet* 2001; **358**: 1389–1399.

95. Lethaby A, Farquhar C, Sarkis A *et al*. Hormone replacement therapy in postmenopausal women: Endometrial hyperplasia and irregular bleeding (Cochrane Review). In: The Cochrane Library, Issue 1, 1999. Oxford: Update Software.

96. Grady D, Gebretsadik T, Kerlikowske K *et al*. Hormone replacement therapy and endometrial cancer risk: A meta-analysis. *Obstet Gynecol* 1995; **85**: 304–313.

97. Pike MC, Peters RK, Cozen W *et al*. Estrogen-progestin replacement therapy and endometrial cancer. *J Natl Cancer Inst* 1997; **89**: 1110–1116.

98. Weiderpass E, Adami H-O, Baron JA *et al*. Risk of endometrial cancer following estrogen replacement with and without progestins. *J Natl Cancer Inst* 1999; **91**: 1131–1137.

99. Weiderpass E, Baron JA, Adami H-O *et al*. Low-potency estrogen and risk of endometrial cancer: A case-control study. *Lancet* 1999; **353**: 1824–1828.

100. Kurman RJ, Moyer DL, Felix JC *et al*. Low doses of norethindrone acetate effectively reduce the incidence of endometrial hyperplasia associated with 1 mg 17 ß estradiol. *Menopause* 1998; **5**: 261.

101. Bjarnason K, Cerin A, Lindgren R *et al*, for the Scandinavian Long Cycle Group. Adverse endometrial effects during long cycle hormone replacement therapy. *Maturitas* 1999; **32**: 161–170.

102. Creasman WT, Henderson D, Hinshaw W *et al*. Estrogen replacement therapy in the patient treated for endometrial cancer. *Obstet Gynecol* 1986; **67**: 326–330.

103. Lee RB, Burke TW, Park RC. Estrogen replacement therapy following treatment for stage I endometrial carcinoma. *Gynecol Oncol* 1990; **36**: 189–191.

104. Chapman JA, DiSaia P, Osann K *et al*. Estrogen replacement in surgical stage I and II endometrial cancer survivors. *Am J Obstet Gynecol* 1996; **175**: 1195–1200.

105. Garg PP, Kerlikowske K, Subak L *et al*. Hormone replacement therapy and the risk of epithelial ovarian carcinoma: A meta-analysis. *Obstet Gynecol* 1998; **92**: 472–479.

106. Bosetti C, Franceschi S, Trichopoulos D *et al*. Relationship between postmenopausal hormone replacement therapy and ovarian cancer. *JAMA* 2001; **285**: 3089–3090.

107. Rodriguez C, Patel AV, Calle EE *et al*. Estrogen replacement therapy and ovarian cancer mortality in a large prospective study of US women. *JAMA* 2001; **285**: 1460–1465.

108. Lacey JV, Mink PJ, Lubin JH *et al*. Menopausal hormone replacement therapy and risk of ovarian cancer. *JAMA* 2002; **288**: 334–342

109. Coughlin SS, Giustozzi A, Smith SJ *et al*. A meta-analysis of estrogen replacement therapy and risk of epithelial ovarian cancer. *J Clin Epidemiol* 2000; **53**: 367–375.

110. Riman T, Dickman PW, Nilsson S *et al*. Hormone replacement therapy and the risk of invasive epithelial ovarian cancer in Swedish women. *J Natl Cancer Inst* 2002; **94**: 497–504.

111. Guidozzi F, Daponte A. Estrogen replacement therapy for ovarian carcinoma survivors: A randomized controlled trial. *Cancer* 1999; **86**: 1013–1018.

112. Burger CE, van Leeuwe, FE, Scheele F *et al*. Hormone replacement therapy in women treated for gynaecological malignancy. *Maturitas* 1999; **32**: 69–76.

113. MacLennan SC, MacLennan AH, Ryan P *et al*. Colorectal cancer and oestrogen replacement therapy. A meta-analysis of epidemiologic studies. *Med J Aust* 1995; **162**: 491–493.

114. Nanda K, Bastian LA, Hasselblad V *et al*. Hormone replacement therapy and risk of colorectal cancer: A meta-analysis. *Obstet Gynecol* 1999; **93**(Suppl): 880–888.

115. Oger E, Scarabin PY. Assessment of risk for venous thromboembolism among users of hormone replacement therapy. *Drugs Aging* 1999; **14**: 55–61.

116. Høibraaten E, Quigstad E, Andersen TO *et al*. The effects of hormone replacement therapy (HRT) on haemostatic variables in women with previous venous thromboembolism — results from a randomized, double-blind clinical trial. *Thromb Haemost* 2001; **85**: 775–781.

117. Miller J, Chan BKS, Nelson HD. Postmenopausal estrogen replacement and risk for venous thromboembolism: a systematic review and meta-analysis for the US Preventative Services Task Force. *Ann Intern Med* 2002; **136**: 680–690.

118. Daly E, Vessey MP, Hawkins MM *et al*. Risk of venous thrombembolism in users of hormone replacement therapy. *Lancet* 1996; **348**: 977–980

119. Jick H, Derby LE, Myers MW *et al*. Risk of hospital admission for idiopathic venous thromboembolism among users of postmenopausal oestrogens. *Lancet* 1996; **348**: 981–983.

120. Pérez Gutthann S, García Rodríguez LA, Castellsague J *et al*. Hormone replacement therapy and risk of venous thromboembolism: population based case-control study. *BMJ* 1997; **314**: 796–800.

121. Grady D, Wenger NK, Herrington D *et al*. Postmenopausal hormone therapy increases the risk for venous thromboembolic disease. The Heart and Estrogen/progestin Replacement Study. *Ann Intern Med* 2000; **132**: 689–696.

122. Varas-Lorenzo C, García Rodríguez LA, Cattaruzzi C *et al*. Hormone replacement therapy and the risk of hospitalization for venous thromboembolism: a population-based study in southern Europe. *Am J Epidemiol* 1998; **147**: 387–390.

123. Effects of estrogen or estrogen/progestin regimens on heart disease risk factors in postmenopausal women. The Postmenopausal Estrogen/Progestin Interventions (PEPI) Trial. The Writing Group for the PEPI trial. *JAMA* 1995; **273**: 199–208.

124. Surgically confirmed gallbladder disease, venous thromboembolism, and breast tumors in relation to postmenopausal estrogen therapy. A report from the Boston Collaborative Drug Surveillance Program. Boston University Medical Center. *N Engl J Med* 1974; **290**: 15–19.

125. Daly E, Vessey MP, Painter R *et al*. Case-control study of venous thromboembolism risk in users of hormone replacement therapy [Letter] *Lancet* 1996; **348**: 1027.

126. Devor M, Barrett-Connor E, Renvall M *et al*. Estrogen replacement therapy and the risk of venous thrombosis. *Am J Med* 1992; **92**: 275–282.

127. Grodstein F, Stampfer MJ, Goldhaber SZ *et al*. Prospective study of exogenous hormones and risk of pulmonary embolism in women. *Lancet* 1996; **348**: 983–987.

128. Cummings SR, Eckert S, Krueger KA *et al.* The effect of raloxifene on risk of breast cancer in postmenopausal women: results from the MORE randomized trial. Multiple Outcomes of Raloxifene Evaluation. *JAMA* 1999; **281**: 2189–2197.

129. Royal College of Obstetricians and Gynaecologists (1999). *Hormone replacement therapy and venous thromboembolism guidelines*. No. 9. London: RCOG.

130. Fanchin R, de Ziegler D, Bergeron C *et al.* Transvaginal administration of progesterone. *Obstet Gynecol* 1997; **90**: 396–401.

Appendix 1 – Drugs

Drug	Trade name	Preparation	Strength	Doses used in menopause	Comments	Side-effects
Oestrogens + progestogens (women with uterus)						
Conjugated oestrogens (equine) + levonorgestrel	Prempak-C 0.625	Tablet	0.625mg (12 tablets) + 75mcg (28 tablets)	MS/OP: 1 conjugated oestrogens tablet/d continuously and 1 levonorgestrel tablet/d from days 17-28 of each treatment cycle	Contraindicated in pregnancy and breast feeding, oestrogen dependent cancer, active thrombophlebitis, thromboembolic disorders or history of recurrent thromboembolism, hepatic disease, Dubin Johnson and Rotor syndromes, undiagnosed vaginal bleeding; caution in migraine, history of breast nodules or fibrocystic disease, uterine fibroids, endometriosis, factors predisposing to thromboembolism; see also norethisterone	Nausea and vomiting, abdominal cramps and bloating, weight changes, breast enlargement and tenderness, premenstrual-like syndrome, sodium and fluid retention, changes in liver function, cholestatic jaundice, altered blood lipids, changes in libido, depression, headache, migraine, dizziness, leg cramps, contact lens irritation; see also norethisterone
	Prempak-C 1.25	Tablet	1.25mg (12 tablets) + 75mcg (28 tablets)			
Conjugated oestrogens (equine) + medroxyprogesterone	Premique	Tablet	0.625mg + 5mg (28 tablets)	MS/OP: 1 tablet/d continuously	Contraindicated in pregnancy and breast feeding, oestrogen dependent cancer, active thromboembolic disorders or history of recurrent	Nausea and vomiting, abdominal cramps and bloating, weight changes, breast enlargement and tenderness, premenstrual-like syndrome, sodium and fluid retention.
	Premique Cycle	Tablet	0.625mg (14 tablets) + 10mg (14 tablets)	MS/OP1 conjugated oestrogens tablet/d for 14 days then 1		

Drug	Trade name	Preparation	Strength	Doses used in menopause	Comments	Side-effects
In USA	Prempro	Tablet	0.625 + 2.5mg (28 tablets) 0.625 +5mg (28 tablets)	medroxyprogesterone tablet for 14 days 1 tablet/d	thromboembolism, hepatic disease, Dubin Johnson and Rotor syndromes, undiagnosed vaginal bleeding; caution in migraine, history of breast nodules or fibrocystic disease, uterine fibroids, endometriosis; factors predisposing to thromboembolism; see also medroxyprogesterone	changes in liver function, cholestatic jaundice, altered blood lipids, changes in libido, depression, headache, migraine, dizziness, leg cramps, contact lens irritation; see also medroxyprogesterone
	Premphase	Tablet:	0.625mg (14 tablets) and 0.625mg +5mg (14 tablets)	1 CEE tablet/d for 14 days and 1 CEE + medroxyprogesterone tablet/d for 14 days		
Oestradiol + dydrogesterone	Femapak 40	Patch + tablet	40mcg/24h (8 patches) + 10mg (14 tablets)	MS: 1 patch twice weekly and 1 tablet/d from days 15-28 of each treatment cycle	Contraindicated in pregnancy and breast feeding, oestrogen dependent cancer, active thrombophlebitis, thromboembolic disorders or history of recurrent thromboembolism, hepatic disease, Dubin Johnson and Rotor syndromes, undiagnosed vaginal bleeding; caution in migraine, history of breast nodules or fibrocystic disease, uterine fibroids, endometriosis; factors predisposing to thromboembolism; continuous combined formulations are not suitable in the perimenopause or within 12 months of last menstrual period; see also dydrogesterone	Nausea and vomiting, abdominal cramps and bloating, weight changes, breast enlargement and tenderness, premenstrual-like syndrome, sodium and fluid retention, changes in liver function, cholestatic jaundice, altered blood lipids, changes in libido, depression, headache, migraine, dizziness, leg cramps, contact lens irritation; transdermal delivery systems (patches) may cause contact sensitization; see also dydrogesterone
	Femapak 80	Patch + tablet	80mcg/24h (8 patches) + 10mg (14 tablets)	MS/OP: 1 patch twice weekly and 1 tablet/d from days 15-28 of each treatment cycle		

Drug	Trade name	Preparation	Strength	Doses used in menopause	Comments	Side-effects
	Femoston 1/10	Tablet	1mg (14 tablets) + 1mg/10mg (14 tablets)	MS/OP: 1 oestradiol tablet/d for 14 days then 1 oestradiol + dydrogesterone tablet/d for 14 days		
	Femoston 2/20	Tablet	2mg (14 tablets) + 2mg/20mg (14 tablets)			
	Femoston Conti	Tablet	1mg + 5mg	MS/OP: 1 tablet/d continuously		
Oestradiol + levonorgestrel	Cyclo-Progynova 1mg	Tablet	1mg (11 tablets) + 1mg/250mcg (10 tablets)	MS: 1 oestradiol tablet/d for 11 days then 1 oestradiol + levonorgestrel tablet/d for 10 days then 7 day interval	Contraindicated in pregnancy and breast feeding, oestrogen dependent cancer, active thrombophlebitis, thromboembolic disorders or history of recurrent thromboembolism, hepatic disease, Dubin Johnson and Rotor syndromes, undiagnosed vaginal bleeding; caution in migraine, history of breast nodules or fibrocystic disease, uterine fibroids, endometriosis, factors predisposing to thromboembolism; see also norethisterone	Nausea and vomiting, abdominal cramps and bloating, weight changes, breast enlargement and tenderness, premenstrual-like syndrome, sodium and fluid retention, changes in liver function, cholestatic jaundice, altered blood lipids, changes in libido, depression, headache, migraine, dizziness, leg cramps, contact lens irritation; transdermal delivery systems (patches) may cause contact sensitization; see also norethisterone
	Cyclo-Progynova 2mg	Tablet	2mg (11 tablets) + 1mg/250mcg (10 tablets)	MS/OP: 1 oestradiol tablet/d for 11 days then 1 oestradiol + levonorgestrel tablet/d for 10 days then 7 day interval		
	Nuvelle	Tablet	2mg (16 tablets) + 75mcg (12 tablets)	MS/OP: 1 oestradiol tablet/d for 16 days then 1 levonorgestrel tablet/d for 12 days		

Drug	Trade name	Preparation	Strength	Doses used in menopause	Comments	Side-effects
	Nuvelle TS	Patch	80mcg/24h (4 patches) + 50mcg/20mcg/24h (4 patches)	MS: 1 oestradiol patch twice weekly for 2 weeks then 1 oestradiol + levonorgestrel patch twice weekly for 2 weeks		
Oestradiol + medroxyprogesterone	Indivina 1mg/2.5mg	Tablet	1mg + 2.5mg	MS/OP: 1 tablet/d continuously	Contraindicated in pregnancy and breast feeding, oestrogen dependent cancer, active thrombophlebitis, thromboembolic disorders or history of recurrent thromboembolism, hepatic disease, Dubin Johnson and Rotor syndromes, undiagnosed vaginal bleeding; caution in migraine, history of breast nodules or fibrocystic disease, uterine fibroids, endometriosis, factors predisposing to thromboembolism; continuous combined formulations are not suitable in the perimenopause or within 12 months of last menstrual period; see also medroxyprogesterone	Nausea and vomiting, abdominal cramps and bloating, weight changes, breast enlargement and tenderness, premenstrual-like syndrome, sodium and fluid retention, changes in liver function, cholestatic jaundice, altered blood lipids, changes in libido, depression, headache, migraine, dizziness, leg cramps, contact lens irritation; transdermal delivery systems (patches) may cause contact sensitization; see also medroxyprogesterone
	Indivina 1mg/5mg	Tablet	1mg + 5mg			
	Indivina 2mg/5mg	Tablet	2mg + 5mg			
	Tridestra	Tablet	2mg (70 tablets) + 2mg/20mg (14 tablets + inactive (7 tablets)	MS/OP: 1 oestradiol tablet/d for 70 days then 1 oestradiol + levonorgestrel tablet/d for 14 days then 1 inactive tablet/d		

Drug	Trade name	Preparation	Strength	Doses used in menopause	Comments	Side-effects
Oestradiol + norethisterone	Adgyn Combi	Tablet	2mg (16 tablets) + 2mg/1mg (12 tablets)	MS: 1 oestradiol tablet/d for 16 days then 1 oestradiol + norethisterone tablet/d for 12 days	Contraindicated in pregnancy and breast feeding, oestrogen dependent cancer, active thrombophlebitis, thromboembolic disorders or history of recurrent thromboembolism, hepatic disease, Dubin Johnson and Rotor syndromes; undiagnosed vaginal bleeding; caution in migraine, history of breast nodules or fibrocystic disease, uterine fibroids, endometriosis, factors predisposing to thromboembolism; continuous combined formulations are not suitable in the perimenopause of within 12 months of last menstrual period; see also norethisterone	Nausea and vomiting, abdominal cramps and bloating, weight changes, breast enlargement and tenderness, premenstrual-like syndrome, sodium and fluid retention, changes in liver function, cholestatic jaundice, altered blood lipids, changes in libido, depression, headache, migraine, dizziness, leg cramps, contact lens irritation; transdermal delivery systems (patches) may cause contact sensitization; see also norethisterone
	Climagest 1mg	Tablet	1mg (16 tablets) + 1mg/1mg (12 tablets)	MS: 1 oestradiol tablet/d for 16 days then 1 oestradiol + norethisterone tablet/d for 12 days		
	Climagest 2mg	Tablet	2mg (16 tablets) + 2mg/1mg (12 tablets)	MS: 1 oestradiol tablet/d for 16 days then 1 oestradiol + norethisterone tablet/d for 12 days		
	Climesse	Tablet	2mg + 1mg	MS/OP: 1 tablet/d continuously		
	Elleste-Duet 1mg	Tablet	1mg (16 tablets) + 1mg/1mg (12 tablets)	MS: 1 oestradiol tablet/d for 16 days then 1 oestradiol + norethisterone tablet/d for 12 days MS/OP: 1 oestradiol tablet/d for 16 days		

Drug	Trade name	Preparation	Strength	Doses used in menopause	Comments	Side-effects
	Elleste-Duet 2mg	Tablet	2mg (16 tablets) + 2mg/1mg (12 tablets)	then 1 oestradiol + norethisterone tablet/d for 12 days		
	Elleste-Duet Conti	Tablet	2mg + 1mg	MS/OP1 tablet/d continuously		
	Estracombi	Patch	50mcg/24h (4 patches) + 50mcg/250mcg/ 24h (4 patches)	MS/OP: 1 oestradiol patch twice weekly for 2 weeks then 1 oestradiol + norethisterone patch twice weekly for 2 weeks		
	Estrapak 50	Patch + tablet	50mcg/24h (8 patches) + 1mg (12 tablets)	MS/OP: 1 oestradiol patch twice weekly continuously and 1 norethisterone tablet/d from days 15-26 of each treatment cycle		
	Evorel Conti	Patch	50mcg/1mg/24h	MS/OP: 1 patch twice weekly continuously		

Drug	Trade name	Preparation	Strength	Doses used in menopause	Comments	Side-effects
	Evorel Pak	Patch + tablet	50mcg/24h (8 patches) + 1mg (12 tablets)	MS/OP: 1 oestradiol patch twice weekly continuously and 1 norethisterone tablet/d from days 15-26 of each treatment cycle		
	Evorel Sequi	Patch	50mcg/24h (4 patches) + 50mcg/170mcg/24h (4 patches)	MS/OP: 1 oestradiol patch twice weekly for 2 weeks then 1 oestradiol + norethisterone patch twice weekly for 2 weeks		
	Kliofem	Tablet	2mg + 1mg	MS/OP: 1 tablet/d continuously		
	Kliovance	Tablet	1mg + 500mcg	MS/OP: 1 tablet/d continuously		
	Nuvelle Continuous	Tablet	2mg + 1mg	MS/OP: 1 tablet/d continuously		
	Trisequens	Tablet				

Drug	Trade name	Preparation	Strength	Doses used in menopause	Comments	Side-effects
	Trisequens Forte	Tablet	2mg (12 tablets) + 2mg/1mg (10 tablets) + 1mg (6 tablets)	MS/OP: 1 oestradiol tablet/d for 12 days then 1 oestradiol + norethisterone tablet/d for 10 days then 1 oestradiol tablet/d for 6 days		
			4mg (12 tablets) + 4mg/1mg (10 tablets) + 1mg (6 tablets)	MS: 1 oestradiol tablet/d for 12 days then 1 oestradiol + norethisterone tablet/d for 10 days then 1 oestradiol tablet/d for 6 days		
In USA	Activella	Tablet	1mg +0.5mg	1 tablet/d continuously		
	Combipatch	Patch	50mcg +140 mcg or 250mcg	1 patch twice weekly		
	FemHRT	Tablet	5mcg ethinyl oestradiol + 1mg	1 tablet/d		
	OrthoPrefest	Tablet	1mg and 1mg + 90mcg	1 of each tablet taken every 3 days continuously		

Drug	Trade name	Preparation	Strength	Doses used in menopause	Comments	Side-effects
Oestrogens (women without uterus)						
Conjugated oestrogens (equine)	Premarin	Tablet	0.625mg, 1.25mg Also available in the USA as 0.3mg, 0.9mg and 2.5mg	MS/OP: 1 tablet/d	Contraindicated in pregnancy and breast feeding, oestrogen dependent cancer, active thrombophlebitis, thromboembolic disorders or history of recurrent thromboembolism, hepatic disease, Dubin Johnson and Rotor syndromes, undiagnosed vaginal bleeding; caution in migraine, history of breast nodules or fibrocystic disease, uterine fibroids, endometriosis, factors predisposing to thromboembolism	Nausea and vomiting, abdominal cramps and bloating, weight changes, breast enlargement and tenderness, premenstrual-like syndrome, sodium and fluid retention, changes in liver function, cholestatic jaundice, altered blood lipids, changes in libido, depression, headache, migraine, dizziness, leg cramps, contact lens irritation
In USA Conjugated oestrogens (synthetic)	Cenestin	Tablet	0.625mg, 0.9mg	1 tablet/d		
Esterified oestrogen	Menest	Tablet	0.3mg, 0.625mg, 1.25mg, 2.5mg			
	Estratab	Tablet	0.3mg, 0.625mg, 2.5mg			
Oestradiol	Adgyn Estro	Tablet	2mg	MS: 2mg/d	Contraindicated in pregnancy and breast feeding, oestrogen dependent cancer, active thrombophlebitis, thromboembolic disorders or history	Nausea and vomiting, abdominal cramps and bloating, weight changes, breast enlargement and tenderness, premenstrual-like syndrome, sodium and
	Aerodiol	Nasal Spray	150mcg/dose	MS: 1-4 sprays/d in divided doses if ≥ 3 sprays		

Drug	Trade name	Preparation	Strength	Doses used in menopause	Comments	Side-effects
	Climaval	Tablet	1mg, 2mg	MS: 1 tablet/d	of recurrent thromboembolism, hepatic disease, Dubin Johnson and Rotor syndromes, undiagnosed vaginal bleeding; caution in migraine, history of breast nodules or fibrocystic disease, uterine fibroids, endometriosis, factors predisposing to thromboembolism	fluid retention, changes in liver function, cholestatic jaundice, altered blood lipids, changes in libido, depression, headache, migraine, dizziness, leg cramps, contact lens irritation; transdermal delivery systems (patches) may cause contact sensitization; nasal spray may cause local irritation, rhinorrhoea and epistaxis
	Dermestril	Patch	25mcg/24h, 50mcg/24h, 100mcg/24h	MS: 1 patch twice weekly		
	Dermestril-Septum	Patch	25mcg/24h, 50mcg/24h, 75mcg/24h	MS: 1 patch weekly		
	Elleste-Solo 1mg	Tablet	1mg	MS: 1mg/d		
	Elleste-Solo 2mg	Tablet	2mg	MS/OP: 12mg/d		
	Elleste-Solo MX 40	Patch	40mcg/24h	MS: 1 patch twice weekly		
	Elleste-Solo MX 80	Patch	80mcg/24h	MS/OP: 1 patch twice weekly		
	Estraderm TTS 25	Patch	25mcg/24h	MS: 1 patch twice weekly		
	Estraderm TTS 25	Patch	50mcg/24h	MS/OP: 1 patch twice weekly		

Drug	Trade name	Preparation	Strength	Doses used in menopause	Comments	Side-effects
	Oestradiol Implants	Implant	25mg, 50mg,100mg	MS/OP: 25-100mg every 4-8 months		
	Evorel	Patch	25mcg/24h	MS: 1 patch twice weekly		
	Evorel	Patch	50mcg/24h, 75mcg/24h, 100mcg/24h	MS/OP: 1 patch twice weekly		
	Fematrix 40	Patch	40mcg/24h	MS: 1 patch twice weekly		
	Fematrix 80	Patch	80mcg/24h	MS/OP: 1 patch twice weekly		
	FemSeven	Patch	50mcg/24h, 75mcg/24h, 100mcg/24h	MS/OP: 1 patch weekly		
	Menorest	Patch	37.5mcg/24h	MS: 1 patch twice weekly		
			50mcg/24h, 75mcg/24h	MS/OP: 1 patch twice weekly		

Drug	Trade name	Preparation	Strength	Doses used in menopause	Comments	Side-effects
	Oestrogel	Gel	0.06%	MS/OP: 2-4 measures/d (1.5-3mg) applied to skin on arm, shoulder or inner thigh		
	Progynova 1mg	Tablet	1mg	MS: 1 mg/d		
	Progynova 2mg	Tablet	2mg	MS/OP: 2mg/d		
	Progynova TS	Patch	50mcg/24h, 75mcg/24h, 100mcg/24h	MS: 1 patch weekly		
	Sandrena	Gel	500mcg/0.5g, 1mg/1g	MP: 0.5-1.5mg/d applied to lower trunk of thighs		
	Zumenon 1mg	Tablet	1mg	MS: 1mg/d		
	Zumenon 2mg	Tablet	2mg	MS/OP: 2mg/d		
Oestradiol + oestriol + estrone	Hormonin	Tablet	600mcg + 270mcg + 1.4mg	MS/OP: 1-2 tablets/d	Contraindicated in pregnancy and breast feeding, oestrogen dependent cancer, active thrombophlebitis, thromboembolic disorders or history of recurrent thromboembolism, hepatic disease; Dubin Johnson and Rotor syndromes, undiagnosed vaginal	Nausea and vomiting, abdominal cramps and bloating, weight changes, breast enlargement and tenderness, premenstrual-like syndrome, sodium and fluid retention, changes in liver function, cholestatic jaundice, altered blood lipids, changes in libido, depression, headache.

Drug	Trade name	Preparation	Strength	Doses used in menopause	Comments	Side-effects
					bleeding; caution in migraine, history of breast nodules or fibrocystic disease, uterine fibroids, endometriosis, factors predisposing to thromboembolism	migraine, dizziness, leg cramps, contact lens irritation
Oestriol	Ovestin	Tablet	1mg	Genitourinary symptoms associated with oestrogen deficiency states: 0.3-3mg/d for 1 month then 0.5-1mg	Contraindicated in pregnancy and breast feeding, oestrogen dependent cancer, active thrombophlebitis, thromboembolic disorders or history of recurrent thromboembolism, hepatic disease, Dubin Johnson and Rotor syndromes, undiagnosed vaginal bleeding; caution in migraine, history of breast nodules or fibrocystic disease, uterine fibroids, endometriosis, factors predisposing to thromboembolism; short term use only	Nausea and vomiting, abdominal cramps and bloating, weight changes, breast enlargement and tenderness, premenstrual-like syndrome, sodium and fluid retention, changes in liver function, cholestatic jaundice, altered blood lipids, changes in libido, depression, headache, migraine, dizziness, leg cramps, contact lens irritation
Estropipate	Harmogen	Tablet	1.5mg	MS/OP: 1.5mg/d; vasomotor symptoms and menopausal vaginitis: up to 3mg/d	Contraindicated in pregnancy and breast feeding, oestrogen dependent cancer, active thrombophlebitis, thromboembolic disorders or history of recurrent thromboembolism, hepatic disease, Dubin Johnson and Rotor syndromes, undiagnosed vaginal bleeding; caution in migraine, history of breast nodules or fibrocystic disease, uterine fibroids, endometriosis, factors predisposing to thromboembolism	Nausea and vomiting, abdominal cramps and bloating, weight changes, breast enlargement and tenderness, premenstrual-like syndrome, sodium and fluid retention, changes in liver function, cholestatic jaundice, altered blood lipids, changes in libido, depression, headache, migraine, dizziness, leg cramps, contact lens irritation

Drug	Trade name	Preparation	Strength	Doses used in menopause	Comments	Side-effects
Progestogens						
Dydrogesterone	Duphaston HRT	Tablet	10mg	MS: 10-20mg/d from days 15-28 of each oestrogen HRT cycle	Contraindicated in hepatic tumours and severe liver impairment, genital warts, breast cancer, severe arterial disease, undiagnosed vaginal bleeding, porphyria; caution in conditions that might worsen with fluid retention (e.g. epilepsy, hypertension, migraine, asthma, cardiac or renal dysfunction), liver impairment, history of depression	Premenstrual-like syndrome (bloating, fluid retention, breast tenderness), weight gain, nausea, headache, dizziness, insomnia, drowsiness, depression, skin reactions
Medroxyprogesterone	Adgyn Medro	Tablet	5mg	MS: 10mg/d from days 15 to 28 of each oestrogen HRT cycle	Contraindicated in hepatic tumours and severe liver impairment, genital warts, breast cancer, severe arterial disease, undiagnosed vaginal bleeding, porphyria, pregnancy; caution in conditions that might worsen with fluid retention (e.g. epilepsy, hypertension, migraine, asthma, cardiac or renal dysfunction), liver impairment, history of depression, breast feeding	Premenstrual-like syndrome (bloating, fluid retention, breast tenderness), weight gain, nausea, headache, dizziness, insomnia, drowsiness, depression, indigestion, skin reactions
	Provera	Tablet	2.5mg, 5mg, 10mg			
In USA Micronized progesterone	Prometrium	Capsule	100mg, 200mg	MS: 200mg/d for 12 continuous days per 28 day cycle	Contraindicated in those with peanut allergy or known sensitivities to peanuts. known or suspected preg-	Dizziness, headache, muscle or bone pain/backpain/joint pain, fatigue, diarrhoea, chest pain, coughing, upper

Drug	Trade name	Preparation	Strength	Doses used in menopause	Comments	Side-effects
					nancy, current or past history of thrombotic disorders, severe liver dysfunction or disease, known or suspected malignancy of breast or reproductive organs, undiagnosed vaginal bleeding, missed abortion, or as a diagnostic test for pregnancy.	respiratory tract infection/viral infection, hot flashes, urinary problems, vaginal discharge/vaginal dryness, night sweats, abdominal pain (cramping), breast pain/breast tenderness, bloating, nausea/vomiting, irritability/mood swings, depression/worry
Norethisterone	Micronor HRT	Tablet	1mg	MS: 1mg/d from days 15 to 26 of each oestrogen HRT cycle	Contraindicated in hepatic tumours and severe liver impairment, genital warts, breast cancer, severe arterial disease, undiagnosed vaginal bleeding, porphyria, pregnancy; caution in conditions that might worsen with fluid retention (e.g. epilepsy, hypertension, migraine, asthma, cardiac or renal dysfunction), liver impairment, history of depression, breast feeding	Premenstrual-like syndrome (bloating, fluid retention, breast tenderness), weight gain, nausea, headache, dizziness, insomnia, drowsiness, depression, skin reactions
Progesterone	Crinone	Vaginal gel	4%	MS: insert 1 applicator full of gel on alternate days on last 12 days of cycle	Contraindicated in hepatic tumours and severe liver impairment, genital warts, breast cancer, severe arterial disease, undiagnosed vaginal bleeding, porphyria; caution in conditions that might worsen with fluid retention (e.g. epilepsy, hypertension, migraine, asthma, cardiac or renal dysfunction), liver impairment, history of depression	Premenstrual-like syndrome (bloating, fluid retention, breast tenderness), weight gain, nausea, headache, dizziness, insomnia, drowsiness, depression, skin reactions

Drug	Trade name	Preparation	Strength	Doses used in menopause	Comments	Side-effects
Androgens						
Testosterone	Testosterone Implant	Implant	100mg, 200mg	MS: 50–100mg implanted every 4-8 months as an adjunct to HRT	Contraindicated in history of primary hepatic tumours, hypercalcaemia, pregnancy, breast feeding, nephrosis; caution in cardiac, renal or hepatic impairment, ischaemic heart disease, hypertension, epilepsy, migraine, diabetes mellitus	Headache, depression, gastrointestinal bleeding, nausea, cholestatic jaundice, anxiety, electrolyte disturbances, androgenic effects
In USA Estrogen + testosterone	Estratest	Tablet	1.25mg esterified estrogen + 2.5 mg methyltestosterone	1 tablet/d cyclically (3 weeks on/1 week off)	Known or suspected pregnancy, lactating women, breast cancer, active thrombophlebitis or thromboembolic disorders, estrogen dependent neoplasia, undiagnosed abnormal genital bleeding and in patients with severe liver damage.	The most commonly reported adverse events are those typical of estrogen therapy (such as breast tenderness, headache, nausea, edema, and abdominal pain) and of androgen treatment (including alopecia, acne, and hirsutism).
	Estratest HS	Tablet	0.625mg esterified estrogen + 1.25 mg methyltestosterone	1-2tablets/d cyclically (3 weeks on/1 week off)		
Other agents						
Raloxifene	Evista	Tablet	60mg	Postmenopausal osteoporosis (prevention and treatment): 60mg/d	Contraindicated in history of venous thromboembolism, undiagnosed uterine bleeding, endometrial cancer, hepatic impairment, cholestasis, severe renal impairment; caution in risk factors for venous	Venous thromboembolism, thrombophlebitis, hot flushes, leg cramps, peripheral oedema, influenza-like symptoms

Drug	Trade name	Preparation	Strength	Doses used in menopause	Comments	Side-effects
					thromboembolism, breast cancer; does not reduce menopausal vasomotor symptoms	
Tibolone	Livial	Tablet	2.5mg	Vasomotor symptoms in oestrogen deficiency, OP. 2.5mg/d	Contraindicated in hormone-dependent tumours, history of cardiovascular or cerebrovascular disease, uninvestigated vaginal bleeding, severe hepatic impairment, pregnancy and breast feeding; caution in renal impairment, history of liver disease, epilepsy, migraine, diabetes mellitus	Weight changes, oedema, dizziness, seborrhoeic dermatitis, vaginal bleeding, headache, abdominal pain, gastrointestinal effects, increased facial hair, depression, arthralgia, myalgia, migraine, visual disturbances, changes in hepatic function, rash, pruritus
Calcitonin						
Calcitonin	Calsynar	Injection	100units/ml; 200units/ml	Postmenopausal osteoporosis: 100units/d with dietary calcium and vitamin D supplements	Caution in history of allergy, renal impairment, heart failure; injections given subcutaneously or intramuscularly	Nausea, vomiting, diarrhoea, flushing, dizziness, tingling of hands, unpleasant taste, rash, abdominal pain, allergic reactions (including anaphylaxis), inflammatory reactions at injection site, nasal spray may cause local irritation and ulceration, rhinitis, sinusitis, epistaxis
	Forcaltonin	Injection	100units/ml			
	Miacalcic	Injection	50units/ml, 100units/ml, 200units/ml			
	Miacalcic	Nasal spray	200units/spray			

Drug	Trade name	Preparation	Strength	Doses used in menopause	Comments	Side-efects
In USA Salmon Calcitonin	Miacalcin	Injection	200I.U./mL	100 I.U. subcutaneous:y every other day		
		Nasal Spray	2200I.U./mL	200I.U./d (1 spray daily in alternate nostrils)		
Bisphosphonates						
Alendronic acid	Fosamax	Tablet	5mg, 10mg	Postmenopausal osteoporosis: 5mg/d (prevention); 10mg/d (treatment)	Contraindicated in oesophageal abnormalities that delay emptying, hypocalcaemia; severe renal impairment; caution in upper gastrointestinal disorders, mild/ moderate renal impairment (reduce dose); swallow whole on an empty stomach (before breakfast) and stand or sit upright for 30min after administration	Oesophageal reactions (oesophagitis, oesophageal ulcers - advise patient to stop treatment if dysphagia, heartburn, pain on swallowing develop); abdominal pain and distension, flatulence, musculoskeletal pain, headache
	Fosamax Once Weekly	M/R tablet	70mg	70mg once weekly (treatment)		
In USA	Fosamax	Tablet	5mg, 10mg, 35mg, 70mg	OS: 10mg/d or 70mg weekly Prevention of OS: 5mg/d or 35mg weekly		
Disodium etidronate + calcium carbonate	Didronel PMO	Tablet	400mg + 1.25g	Postmenopausal osteoporosis (prevention and treatment): 1 disodium etidronate tablet/d for 14 days then 1 calcium	Contraindicated in moderate to severe renal impairment; caution in mild renal impairment (reduce dose); conditions associated with hypercalcaemia and hypercalciuria; avoid food (especially products containing calcium), iron, mineral	Nausea, diarrhoea, constipation, abdominal pain, asymptomatic hypocalcaemia

Drug	Trade name	Preparation	Strength	Doses used in menopause	Comments	Side-effects
				carbonate tablet/d for 76 days	supplements and antacids for at least 2h before and after treatment	Gastrointestinal effects (dyspepsia, nausea, diarrhoea, constipation, oesophageal stricture, duodenitis), headache, musculoskeletal pain
Risedronate sodium	Actonel	Tablet	5mg	Postmenopausal osteoporosis (prevention and treatment): 5mg/d	Contraindicated in hypocalcaemia, severe renal impairment; caution in oesophageal abnormalities that delay emptying, renal impairment; mild/moderate renal impairment (reduce dose); swallow whole on an empty stomach (before breakfast) and stand or sit upright for 30min after administration	
In USA Risedronate	Actonel	Tablet	5mg, 35mg			

Key: MS menopausal symptoms; OP osteoporosis prophylaxis

Appendix 2 – Useful Addresses and Websites

Comprehensive overview of a broad variety of health care topics for women
http://www.nlm.nih.gov/medlineplus/menopause.html

European Menopause and Andropause Society
http://emas.obgyn.net/
(Position paper of EMAS, results from WHI and HERS II - implications for women and the prescriber of HRT) *Maturitas* 2002; **42**: 255–258)

National Institute of Aging: educational material for women (also contains postal addresses of societies, institutions and foundations focusing on women's health care issues)
http://www.nia.nih.gov/health/pubs/menopause/menopause.pdf

National Womens' Health Information Centre
http://www.4women.org/

National Cancer Institute — Postmenopausal hormone use
http://www.cancer.gov/ClinicalTrials/digest-postmenopausal-hormone-use

Report of NAMS Advisory Panel on Postmenopausal Hormone therapy (considering the results of the HERS and WHI trial)
http://www.menopause.org/news.html/advisory

Suggested alternative therapies to HRT
http://nccam.nih.gov/health/alerts/menopause/

Women's Health Initiative
http://www.nhlbi.nih.gov/whi/index.html

Index

Since the major subject of this book is the menopause, entries have been kept to a minimum under this term: readers are advised to seek more specific entries.

Page numbers followed by 'f' indicate figures: page numbers followed by 't' indicate tables.

This index is in letter-by-letter order, whereby spaces and hyphens in main entries are excluded from the alphabetization process.

Abbreviations used in the index are as on (vi)

A

Addison's disease 13
adrenal gland dysfunction,
  hot flushes 105–106
aging signs, frequently
  asked questions
  104–105
alcohol consumption
  breast cancer 81
  non-oral oestrogen
    replacement therapy 33
alendronate
  characteristics 137
  fracture prevention 63t
  osteoporosis prevention 62
alpha oestrogens 95
Alzheimer's disease
  prevention
  frequently asked questions
    103
  HRT 76–77
amenorrhoea 13
  menopause diagnosis 9
  premature menopause 17
American Association of
  Clinical Endo-
  crinologists (AACE)
  diagnosis guidelines 15
  menopause management
    guidelines 92
American Heart Association
  (AHA), HRT

  recommendations
    69–73, 69t
androgen deficiency 43–44
  oestrogen therapy 44
  signs/symptoms 44, 44t, 46
androgen replacement
  therapy 41–50
  algorithm 46t
  dose 47
  oestrogen combination 48f,
    121–122, 122–123,
    135
    CVD prevention 68t
    osteoporosis prevention
      60
  risks 48t
  routes of administration 47,
    49, 50t
  types used 49–50
androgens
  changes 13
  measurement 41, 43
  menopause diagnosis 16
androstenedione changes
  42t
angiotensinogen, oestrogen
  effects 31
arthritis, menopause
  diagnosis 15
atherosclerosis, HRT clinical
  trial 67, 69
autoimmune diseases 13

B

benign breast disease 81–82
biochanin A 94
bisphosphonates
  characteristics 137–138
  fracture prevention 63t
  osteoporosis prevention 62,
    105
    HRT combination 60
  randomized controlled trials
    62, 63t
  side effects 62
bladder training 22
bleeding problems
  continuous HRT 39
  cyclical HRT 38–39
bloating 35
blood pressure (BP) 40
body mass index (BMI) 15
bone density
  age-related changes 52f
  dual x-ray absorptiometry
    measurement 54–55,
    56–57f
  fracture risk 54–55
  raloxifene effects 63
bone structure 52f
breast cancer 78–84
  alcohol consumption 81
  benign breast disease 81–82
  family history 84
  frequently asked questions
    102
  HRT 79, 81–84, 82t
    CEE/MPA combination
      therapy 82
    CEE therapy 82
    mortality 83
    oestrogen/progesterone
      combination therapy
      82–83
    oestrogen/progestin
      combination therapy 83
  incidence 78f, 80f, 80t
  Iowa Women's Health
    Study 81

  NHANES 1
    epidemiological Follow
      Up Study 81
  lifetime risk 78
  meta-analysis 81–82
  Nurses Health Study 82
  oestrogen effects 78–79
  survivors 83–84
Breast Cancer Detection
    Demonstration Project
    82–83
breast disease, benign
    81–82
breast examinations
  frequently asked questions
    103–104
  menopause diagnosis 15

C

calcitonin
  characteristics 136–137
  fracture prevention 63t
  randomized controlled trial
    63t
calcium supplements
  frequently asked questions
    103
  osteoporosis prevention 62,
    105
  randomized controlled trial
    59t
cancer 78–88
  see also individual cancers
cardiovascular disease
    (CVD) 10
  HRT 40, 64–75
    clinical trials 65–69
    recommendations 69–73,
      69t
    see also HERS; Women's
      Health Initiative (WHI)
      trial
  mortality 64f
  prevention
    clinical trials 73
    raloxifene 73

cervical cancer, HRT
    contraindications 88
chemotherapy, premature
    menopause 14
cholesterol 70
    HRT effect 65
chromosome analysis 17
clonidine 21
cognitive impairment, HRT
    76–77
Colles fracture 51
colorectal cancer
    frequently asked questions
        102
    HRT 88
    Women's Health Initiative
        trial 88
complementary therapies
    104
complications (of
    menopause) 10, iii
    see also specific
        diseases/disorders
conjugated equine
    oestrogens (CEE)
    therapy 30t, 128
    atherosclerosis protection
        67, 69
    breast cancer risk 82
    clinical trials 58–59t, 67,
        68t, 69, 74
    component development
        95–96
    compounds used 120–121
    CVD prevention 64–65,
        65–67
    hot flush therapy 20–21
    levonorgestrel combination
        120
    medroxyprogesterone
        combination 120–121
    MPA combination
        atherosclerosis protection
            67, 69
        breast cancer risk 82
        clinical trials 67, 68t

colorectal cancer risk 88
CVD prevention 71, 73
endometrial hyperplasia
    risk 85–86
osteoporosis prevention 60
pharmacokinetics 32f
progesterone combination
    85–86
stroke risk 74
contraception, frequently
    asked questions 101
coronary artery bypass
    grafting (CABG) 72t
coronary heart disease
    (CHD)
    HRT effects 66f
    Women's Health Initiative
        trial 71, 72t, 73
corticosteroid therapy,
    androgen insufficiency
    44
cortisol-binding protein,
    oestrogen effects 31
coumestans 94
coumestrol 94
cyproterone acetate 36t
    randomized controlled trial
        59t
cystitis iii

D
daidzein 94
definition (of menopause)
    9t
dehydroepiandrosterone
    sulphate (DHEAS)
    age-related decline 41
    changes 42t
    menopause diagnosis 16
    oral replacement 50t
    radioimmunoassay 41
dementia, HRT 76, 77
depression 29
    frequently asked questions
        102
desogestrel 36t

diabetes mellitus
  frequently asked questions
    104
  hot flushes 105–106
  HRT 40
  non-oral oestrogen
    replacement therapy 34
  premature menopause 13
**diagnosis (of menopause)
  9, 15–17**
  frequently asked questions
    100, 102
  hormonal evaluation 16
  medical history 15
dietary history 15
Dong Quai 22
Dowager's Hump 54
drug interactions, HRT 35
**dual x-ray absorptiometry
  (DEXA)**
  bone density measurement
    54–55, 56–57f
  patient groups 55
dydrogesterone 36, 36t
  as HRT 133
  oestradiol combination
    121–122
dyspareunia 25–26, iii
  frequently asked questions
    101
  treatment 26–27
  vaginal atrophy 23

E
**emotional/psychological
  symptoms 28–29, 28t**
  contributory factors 28t
  treatment 29
endometrial atrophy 94–95
endometrial cancer 84–85
  frequently asked questions
    106
  HRT 85, 86–87
  oestrogen/progestogen
    combination therapy
    84–85

  oestrogen replacement
    therapy 84
  risk factors 84–85
  Women's Health Initiative
    trial 85
**endometrial hyperplasia
  85–87**
  CEE/MPA combination
    therapy 85–86
  CEE/progesterone
    combination therapy
    85–86
  HRT regimen differences 85,
    86
  norethisterone/oestradiol
    combination therapy
    86
  oestrogen replacement
    therapy 84
  progestogen replacement
    therapy 35, 86
**epithelial pallor, vaginal
  atrophy 24**
estrogen *see* **oestrogen**
estrone, in HRT 131–132
estropipate, in HRT 132
ethynyl oestradiol 30t
etidronate
  characteristics 137–138
  fracture prevention 63t
  randomized controlled trial
    63t
**European Menopause and
  Andropause Society
  139**
**evening primrose rose oil
  22**
**exercise, osteoporosis
  prevention 62**

F
**family history, breast cancer
  84**
**female androgen
  insufficiency** *see*
  androgen deficiency

fluoride, osteoporosis
   prevention 60
fluorinated testosterone 49
follicle stimulating hormone
   (FSH)
   changes 11, 12f
   frequently asked questions
      100
   menopause diagnosis 16
   premature menopause 13,
      17
formication 20
formononetin 94
fractures
   common sites 53f
   frequently asked questions
      102
   HRT effects 58–59
   prevalence 54
   prevention 63t
      clinical trials 63t
   risk 54–55
      bone density 54–55
      raloxifene effects 63
   see also osteoporosis;
      specific fractures
frequently asked questions
      100–106
   aging signs 104–105
   Alzheimer's disease 103
   breast cancer 102
   breast examinations
      103–104
   breast size 101
   calcium supplements 103
   complementary therapies
      104
   contraception 101
   diabetes mellitus 104
   diagnosis 100, 102
   dyspareunia 101
   endometrial cancer 106
   FSH levels 100
   hot flushes 100, 104,
      105–106
   HRT 101–106

   HRT duration 101–102
   migraines 106
   myocardial infarction 104
   oral contraceptives 106
   osteoporosis 103, 105
   sexual dysfunction 101
   skin effects 101
   symptoms 100, 102
   urinary incontinence 103
   uterine fibroids 104
   vertebral fracture 105
   weight gain 103
friability, vaginal atrophy
   24

G
gels
   HRT 96
   testosterone replacement
      therapy 49, 50t
genistein 94

H
HERS trial 64–65
   cognitive impairment 76–77
   CVD 66f, 70
   lipid profile effects 67f
   progestogen therapy 73
   stroke data 74
   VTE 91–92
high-density lipoprotein
   (HDL) 70, 73
   HRT effects 66f
hip fractures 51
hormone levels 11–13, 11t
   menopause diagnosis 16
   postmenopause 42t, 43f
   premature menopause
      diagnosis 17
   premenopause 42t, 43f
hormone replacement
   therapy (HRT) 30–40,
   iii
   agents used 30–40
   bone density effects 60
   breast cancer 79, 81

incidence 81
  risk factor 79, 81–84, 82t
  survivors 83–84
colorectal cancer 88
compliance 40
compounds used 120–135
contraindications 35t
  cervical cancer 88
  endometrial cancer
    86–87
delivery system development
    96
dosing 39–40
duration
  frequently asked questions
    101–102
  osteoporosis prevention
    60
dyspareunia treatment 26
endometrial protection 37t
fracture prevention 58–59,
    63t
frequently asked questions
    101–106
gels 96
hot flush treatment 20–21
indications 39–40
monitoring 40
nasal spray 96
oophorectomy 47
osteoporosis prevention
    60–61
  risks/benefits 61t
patient lifestyle 70
post-endometrial cancer
    86–87
post ovarian cancer 87–88
post VTE 92
psychological symptoms
    therapy 29
regimens 37–38
  bleed-free 94
  combined 48f, 60, 85, 94
  continuous 37t, 38, 39,
    85, 94
  cyclical 37t, 38–39

endometrial cancer risk
    85
  endometrial hyperplasia
    risk 85, 86
  osteoporosis prevention
    60
  ovarian cancer risk 87
  sequential 85, 86
as risk factor
  endometrial hyperplasia
    85–87
  ovarian cancer 87–88
  VTE 89–92
sexual dysfunction treatment
    26–27
side effects 40, iii
  bleeding problems 38–39
uptake 30t
urinary incontinence therapy
    22–23
urinary tract infection
    therapy 23, 24f
vaginal atrophy treatment
    26–27
see also specific hormones
hot flushes 19–22, iii
adrenal gland dysfunction
    105–106
aetiology 19
  non-hormonal causes
    105–106
complications 20
definition 19
diabetes mellitus 105–106
frequently asked questions
    100, 104, 105–106
HRT therapy 39
psychological factors 28
raloxifene side effects 62
severity 19–20
treatment 20–22
trigger factors 20
**β-human chorionic gonado-
    trophin, menopause
    diagnosis 17**
hyperandrogenism 16, 43

hypercholesterolaemia 33
hyperprolactinaemia 16
hypertension 33
hypertriglyceridaemia 34
hypothyroidism 13
hysterectomy 12, 94–95
    ovarian failure 14

I
insomnia 28, iii
intrauterine devices (IUDs)
    progesterone delivery
        systems 98
    progestogen replacement
        therapy 37
Iowa Women's Health Study
    81
isoflavones 94

K
KY jelly 25
kyphosis 54

L
levonorgestrel 36t
    CEE combination 120
    oestradiol combination
        122–123
life expectancy 9, 10f
lignans 94
lipid profile 65, 66f
low-density lipoprotein
    (LDL) 70
    HRT effect 65, 66f
lutenizing hormone (LH)
    changes 11, 12f
    menopause diagnosis 16
    premature menopause 13

M
malabsorption 33
mammography 40
management (of menopause)
    American Association of
        Clinical Endocrinologists
        guidelines 92

drugs used 120–138
future work 93–99
HRT see hormone
        replacement therapy
        (HRT)
Royal College of Obstetrician
        and Gynaecologists
        guidelines 92, 92t

mastalgia 35, 40
medical history, menopause
    diagnosis 15
medroxyprogesterone
    acetate (MPA) therapy
    36, 36t
    androgenic effects 36
    CEE combination 120–121
        breast cancer risk 82
        colorectal cancer risk 88
        endometrial hyperplasia
            risk 85–86
    clinical trials 58t, 59t, 68t,
        74
    CVD prevention 64–65
    hot flush therapy 20–21
    as HRT 133
    oestradiol combination 123
    oestrogen combination 68t
    stroke risk 74
megestrol acetate 21
mestranolol 58t
methyltestosterone 49, 50t
micturition
    frequency iii
    pain 22
migraines
    frequently asked questions
        106
    non-oral oestrogen
        replacement therapy 34
Multiple Outcomes of
    Raloxifene Evaluation
    (MORE) trial 73
    VTE 92
mumps virus infection,
    premature menopause
    13

myocardial infarction (MI)
frequently asked questions
104
HRT effects 66f
morbidity/mortality 71f

N
nandrolone decenoate 50t
nasal spray
HRT 96
oestrogen therapy 33, 34
**National Cancer Institute
139**
**National Institute of Aging
139**
**National Women's' Health
Information Centre
139**
nausea 35
**NHANES 1 epidemiological
follow Up Study 81**
night sweats 20
norethisterone 36, 36t
as HRT 134
oestradiol combination
124–127
endometrial hyperplasia
risk 86
norgestimate 36t
Nurses Health Study
breast cancer risk 82
CVD 70–71

O
oestradiol
changes 42t
premenopause 11
**oestradiol therapy 31,
128–131**
clinical trial 59t
clinical trials 58t
delivery systems 96
dydrogesterone combination
121–122
levonorgestrel combination
122–123

medroxyprogesterone
combination 123
norethisterone combination
124–127
endometrial hyperplasia
risk 86
oestriol and estrone
combination 131–132
oophorectomy 47
osteoporosis prevention 60
transdermal 58t
17β-oestradiol therapy 30t
osteoporosis prevention 60
substitute development 95
oestriol therapy 132
oestradiol and estrone
combination 131–132
oestrogen 9
breast cancer 78–79
changes 11
component development
95–96
oophorectomy 13, 14f
perimenopause 16
pharmacological
development 98–99
premature menopause 13
oestrogen receptors
age-related changes 70
methylation 70
psychological symptoms 28
**oestrogen replacement
therapy 30–35**
androgen combination 48f,
121–122, 122–123,
123, 135
CVD prevention 68t
osteoporosis prevention
60
androgen insufficiency 44
compounds used 120–132
contraindications 35, 35t
CVD prevention 65, 68t
results 68t
drug interactions 35
endometrial cancer risk 84

endometrial hyperplasia risk
84
metabolism 31
affecting factors 32t
monotherapy 94
oral 31
metabolic effects 32t
side effects 31
tissue concentrations 34t
urinary tract infection
therapy 23
osteoporosis prevention 60
ovarian cancer risk 87
pharmacokinetics 31, 32f,
33
progesterone combination
82–83
progestin combination 87
progestogen combination
83, 84–85
routes of administration
30–31, 31t, 33
clinical implications
33–34
intravaginal 23
nasal spray 33, 34
non-oral 33–34
oral see above
slow release 33
topical 33
transdermal 23, 24
side effects 34–35
variation 34–35
testosterone combination
135
types used 30t
urinary tract infection
therapy 23
vaginal atrophy therapy 24
VTE risk 89–92, 90f
meta-analysis 91f

oestrone
changes 11, 42t
premenopause 11
oophorectomy
androgen deficiency 41, 43

hormone levels 42t
HRT 47
oestrogen levels 14, 14f
ovarian cancer therapy
87–88
premature menopause 13
sexual dysfunction 27
oral contraceptives 9
androgen insufficiency 44
frequently asked questions
106
perimenopause 16
osteoporosis 10, 51–63, iii
definition 51
frequently asked questions
103, 105
menopause diagnosis 15
morbidity/mortality 54, 54f
oophorectomy 13
prevention 62
future work 98–99
HRT 60–61
non-hormonal 105
selective estrogen receptor
modulators 61–62
risk factors 55t
signs/symptoms 54
see also fractures
ovarian cancer
HRT 87–88
as risk factor 87–88
incidence 87
premature menopause
87–88
prevalence 87
therapy 87–88
ovarian failure 13
hysterectomy 14

P
palpitations 20, iii
**parathyroid hormone (PTH)
63t**
peak bone mass 51
pelvic examination 15
pelvic floor exercises 22

PEPI trial *see*
Postmenopausal
Estrogen/Progestin
Interventions (PEPI)
trial
perimenopause
definition 9t
FSH levels 11
hormone levels 12f, 16
oral contraceptives 16
petechiae 24
pharmacokinetics,
oestrogen therapy
31, 32f, 33
phenytoin, oestrogen
interactions 35
physical examination 15
phytoestrogens
menopause management
93–94
osteoporosis prevention 61
pituitary adrenal
insufficiency 44
Postmenopausal
Estrogen/Progestin
Interventions (PEPI)
trial
hot flush therapy 20–21
osteoporosis prevention 61
progestogen replacement
therapy 35
psychological symptoms
therapy 29
venous thromboembolism
risk 89
postmenopause
definition 9t
hormone levels 12f, 42t, 43f
sex hormone binding
globulin 41
posture, menopause
diagnosis 15
premature menopause
13–14
aetiology 13
chemotherapy 14

ovarian cancer 87–88
radiotherapy 14
surgery 13–14
diagnosis 12, 17
hormone changes 13
symptoms 13
premenopause hormone
levels 11, 12f, 42t,
43f
progesterone
changes 11
component development
97–98
menopause diagnosis 16
progesterone replacement
therapy 133–134,
134
oestrogen combination
82–83
routes of administration 98
micronized 133–134
oral delivery 97–98
progestin, oestrogen
combination 83
progestin replacement
therapy, oestrogen
combination 87
progestogen component
development 97–98
progestogen replacement
therapy 35–37
clinical trials 35
compounds used 133–135
CVD prevention 73
endometrial hyperplasia risk
86
hot flush therapy 20–21
metabolism 36
oestrogen combination
84–85
routes of administration 37
IUD 37
micronized 20–21
topical 37
side effects 36–37
substances used 36t

tibolone 37
prolactin, menopause diagnosis 16
psychosexual counselling 27

Q
quality of life assessment 15

R
race 9
peak bone mass 51
venous thromboembolism risk 91
radioimmunoassay, DHEAS 41
radiotherapy, premature menopause 14
raloxifene
bone density effects 63
characteristics 135–136
clinical trial 73
CVD prevention 73
fracture prevention 63t
osteoporosis prevention 61–62, 105
psychological symptoms therapy 29
randomized controlled trial 63t
side effects 62
VTE risk 92
randomized controlled trials (RCTs)
alendronate 63t
bisphosphonates 62, 63t
calcitonin 63t
calcium supplements 59t
etidronate 63t
fracture prevention 63t
HRT 58–59t
conjugated equine oestrogens 58t, 59t
cyproterone acetate 59t
dementia prevention 77

fracture prevention 63t
medroxyprogesterone acetate 58t, 59t
oestradiol valerate 59t
mestranolol 58t
parathyroid hormone 63t
raloxifene 63t
risedronate 63t
vitamin D supplementation 59t, 63t
Replens 25
risedronate
characteristics 138
fracture prevention 63t
osteoporosis prevention 62
randomized controlled trial 63t
Royal College of Obstetrician and Gynaecologists, management guidelines 92, 92t

S
selective estrogen receptor modulators (SERMs) 93
osteoporosis prevention 61–62
selective steroid receptor modulators 93
sex hormone binding globulin (SHBG)
changes 13
oestrogen effects 31
post menopause 41
sexual dysfunction 25–27
cycle 25f
frequently asked questions 101
non-hormonal factors 26t
signs/symptoms 25–26
testosterone levels 45t
treatment 26–27
sexual history 15
Short Personal Experiences

Questionnaire 26
smoking 9
  cessation 62
statins 65
stress incontinence 23
  frequently asked questions
    103
stroke
  HRT 74
  prevention 74
  Women's Health Initiative
    trial 71, 72t, 73
symptoms (of menopause)
    10f, 18–29, iii
  frequently asked questions
    100, 102
  incidence 18
  severity 18, 19f
  summary 18f
  see also specific symptoms

T
testosterone
  assays 41, 43
  changes 42t, 43f
  menopause diagnosis 16
testosterone cyprionate
    50t
testosterone enanthate 50t
testosterone replacement
    therapy 47, 135
  oestrogen combination 135
  oophorectomy 47
  oral micronized 49
  routes of administration 49,
    50t
  sexual dysfunction treatment
    27
  types used 49, 50t
testosterone undecenoate
    50t
thyroid dysfunction, hot
    flushes 105–106
thyroid hormones, meno-
    pause diagnosis 16
tibolone

characteristics 136
  osteoporosis prevention 60
transdermal patches
  oestradiol 58t
  testosterone 49, 50t
trigger factors, hot flushes
    20
triglycerides
  HRT effect 66f
  oestrogen effects 31
Turner's syndrome 13

U
ultrasound, bone density
    measurement 54–55
unstable angina
  HERS trial 70
  HRT clinical trial 69
  morbidity/mortality 71f
urge incontinence 23
urinary incontinence 22–23
  frequently asked questions
    103
  treatment 22–23
urinary tract infections
    (UTIs) 23
  treatment 23, 24f
uterine fibroids 104

V
vaginal atrophy 23–25
  aetiology 23
  dyspareunia 23
  HRT therapy 39
  signs/symptoms 23–24, 24f
  treatment 24–25
vaginal dryness 23, iii
vaginal moisturizers 25
venous thromboembolism
    (VTE)
  HERS 91–92
  high-risk patients 91–92
  HRT 40, 92
    as risk factor 89–92, 90f
  MORE 92
  pathophysiology 89

prophylaxis 69t
risk factors
  HRT 89–92
  oestrogen replacement
    therapy 89–92, 90f
  race 91
  raloxifene 92
  Women's Health Initiative
    trial 72t, 90
vertebral fractures
frequently asked questions
  105
prevalence 53f
vitamin D supplementation
fracture prevention 63t
frequently asked questions
  103
osteoporosis prevention 105
randomized controlled trial
  59t, 63t
**vitamin E supplementation
  22**

W
weight gain
frequently asked questions
  103
HRT side effects 35
WHI trial *see* **Women's
  Health Initiative (WHI)
  trial**
WISDOM *see* **Women's
  International Study of
  Long Duration
  Oestrogen for
  Menopause (WISDOM)**
**women's health care centres
  iii**
**Women's Health Initiative-
  Memory Study
  (WHIMS) 77**
**Women's Health Initiative
  (WHI) trial 39, 65,
  67, 139**
colorectal cancer risk 88
CVD effects 71, 72f, 72t, 73

discontinuation 65
endometrial cancer risks 85
results 68t
stroke risk 74
VTE risk 90
**Women's International
  Study of Long
  Duration Oestrogen
  for Menopause
  (WISDOM)**
discontinuation 67
HRT prevention of dementia
  77
**World Health Organization,
  osteoporosis
  definition 51**